**You are what you eat.
Unless you're pregnant.**

Colofon

Author	Pascal Rotteveel
Concept	Pascal Rotteveel
	www.pascalrotteveel.com
Photography	Rene Mesman
	www.renemesman.nl
Foodstyling	Claartje Lindhout
	www.claartjelindhout.com
Retouching	Luminous-ci
	www.luminous-ci.com
Copy editing	John Louhglin
Copy editing	Het Vertaalcollectief
	www.hetvertaalcollectief.nl
Design	Dennis van Gaalen & Pascal Rotteveel
	www.dennisvangaalen.nl

BISPUBLISHERS

Building Het Sieraad
Postjesweg 1
1057 DT Amsterdam
The Netherlands
T +31 (0)20 515 02 30
bis@bispublishers.com
www.bispublishers.com

ISBN 978 90 6369 548 4

Pregnancy Cookbook

by Pascal Rotteveel

Before you
dig in

Ever since my sister got pregnant for the first time I have been intrigued with how a pregnancy can alter the tastebuds of a woman. Four healthy nephews later it had gotten so that the first thing I would ask my expecting friends and family was, "What's the weirdest thing you crave?". The answers were every now and then so disturbingly awesome, that I felt the need to immortalise them properly. Together with the talented René Mesman and Claartje Lindhout we translated the recipes found through friends, family, and the internet into iconic images.

The book is created with the struggle of pregnancy cravings in mind. It's intention is to pay homage to the crazy pregnancy cravings, and find the quickest way to satisfaction. It's not some food snob's cookbook with detailed recipes down to the milligram but more the broad strokes to unconventional cravings. See this book as an exploration of culinary wonder and (let's be honest) disgust, with some tips and tricks to get your hands on these tasty snacks ASAP.

Besides my ability to make a mean risotto, I know very little about cooking, and let alone recipes. In no way should this book be perceived as a dietary guide.

Crave carefully.

Embrace
the crave

Caramerring

Ingredients

Rollmops

Salted
caramel

This dish looks like it has been invented by a peg legged pirate with a sweet tooth, but nothing could be further from the truth. This recipe comes straight out of the guilty pleasure galley of pregnant landlubbers.

It tastes way better than it looks, and it's certainly one of the most disturbing I've encountered. But if it scratches your itch, who am I to judge?

Take some rollmop herrings and lay them on a plate. Melt some salted caramel, and pour it over them. If you wait a little, the caramel will coagulate and have more of a bite, or you can just eat it while it's still warm. Don't burn your tongue, though: melted caramel can be extremely hot.

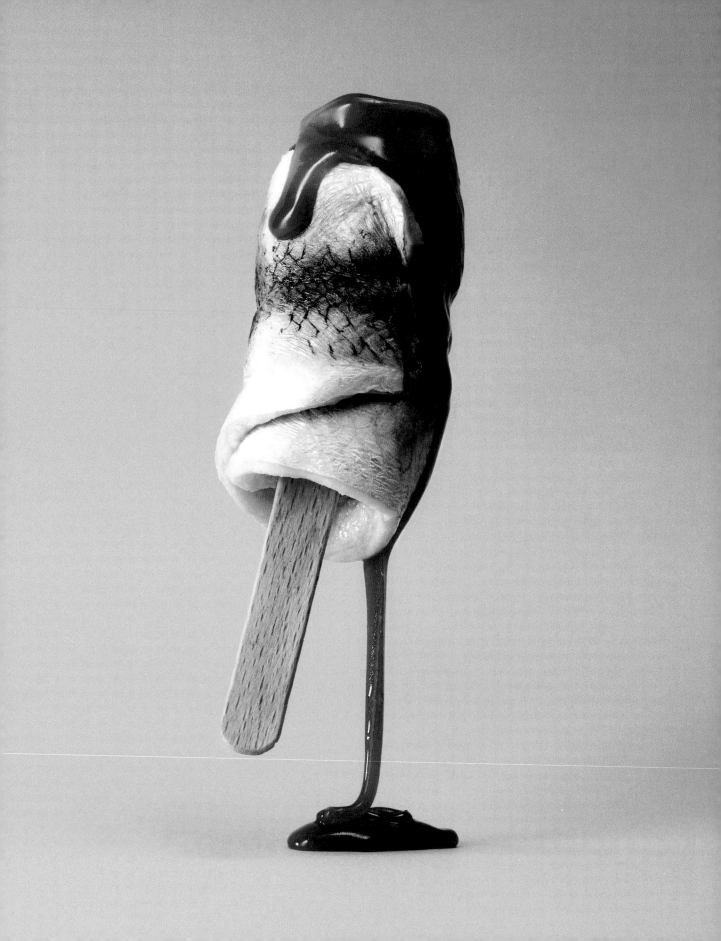

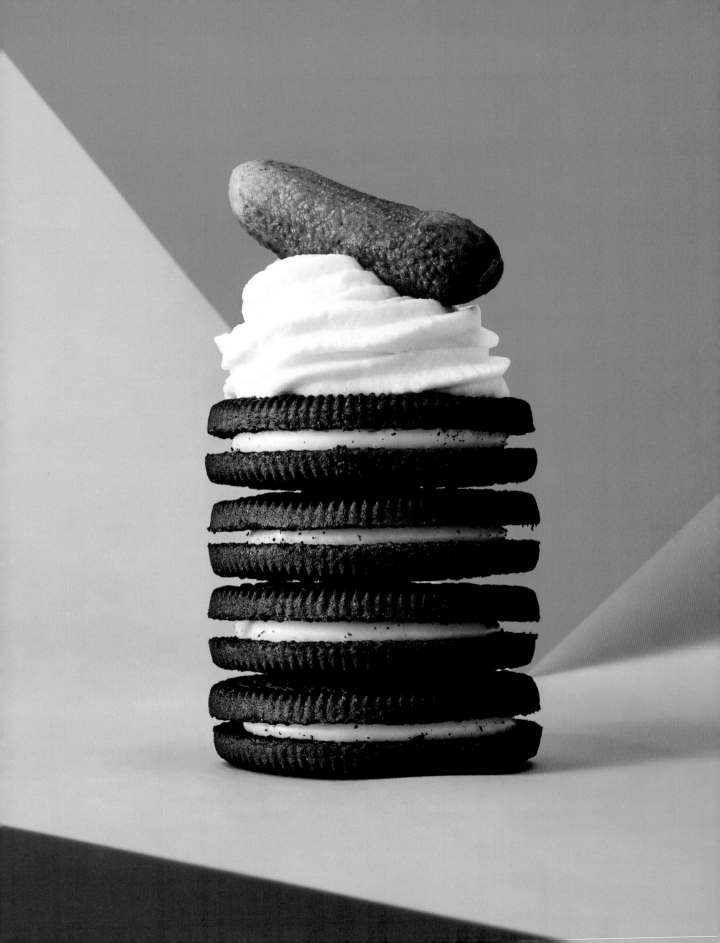

Pickloreo

Ingredients

Oreo cookies

Pickles

Whipped cream

A recipe that has upset and excited many people. Some see the Oreo as the holiest of holies, a cookie not to be tinkered with, others as a blank canvas of opportunity, a springboard of flavor waiting to catapult you into ecstasy. As you can probably guess, by "others" I mean "pregnant women".

You're about to discover the Pickloreo, a cookie and pickle sandwich with sweet cream on top. Or in the middle. Or on the bottom. Whatever tickles your fancy. Unlike the recipes you've seen so far, this one requires a little bit of prep, but that's half the fun of eating.

Disassemble each Oreo into three parts: cookie, cream, cookie. Slice up some pickles, two slices for each sandwich. Stack the Pickloreo in the following order: cookie, pickle, sweet, sweet delicious cream, pickle, cookie. Make sure you build plenty so you can out-eat your craving without having to build refills. So stack your stacks on stacks.

Brown Salami

Ingredients

2 Tablets of Dark or
Milk Chocolate

One Firm Fennel Salami

Unlike the header might suggest, this is not the title of a bad porno, this is literally chocolate covered Salami. So no bad moustaches or poorly written plumbing scenarios. However, this scenario will end in a climax. Because the sweetness of the chocolate and the saltiness of the Salami are, apparently, a foodgasm.

Depending on your preference you can either melt some dark or milk chocolate au bain-marie but a microwave will do fine too. Once it is melted, poor it directly on the salami because it will settle quite fast, a good thing for the salami, a bad thing for your bowl.

If you've got a deep throat or if you're just in need of a hasty snack, you can always just squeeze some salami in between two bricks of chocolate and turn it into a chocolate salami sub. The satisfaction won't be lesser for it.

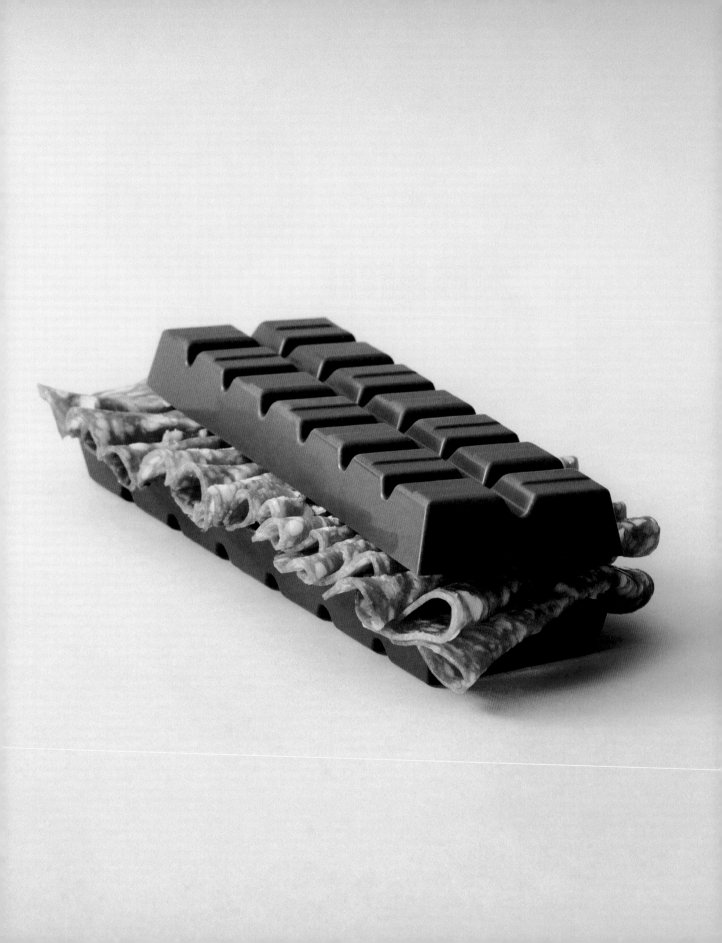

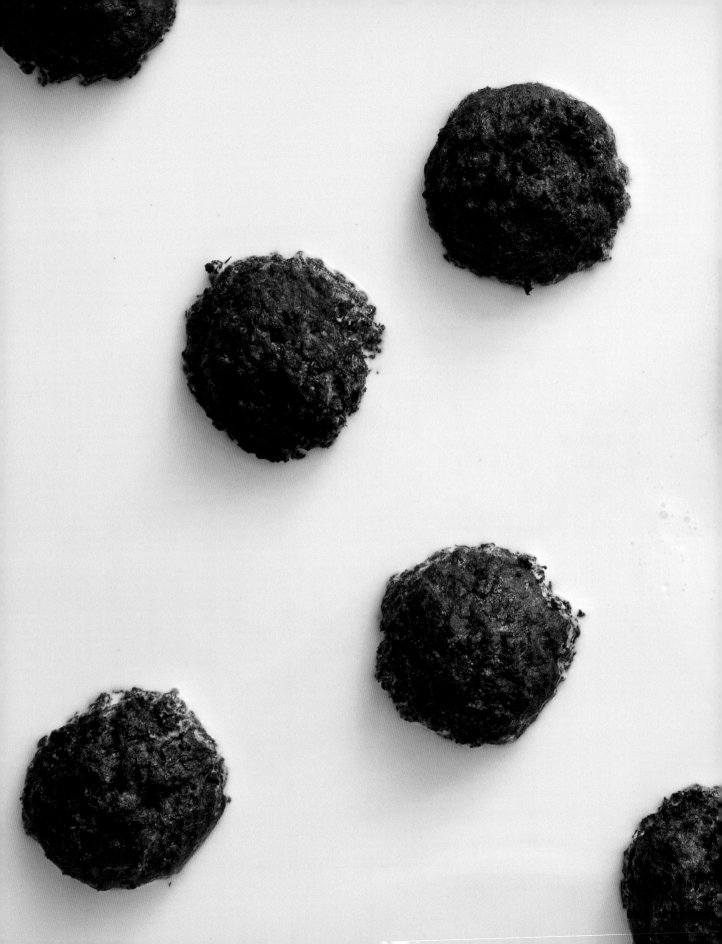

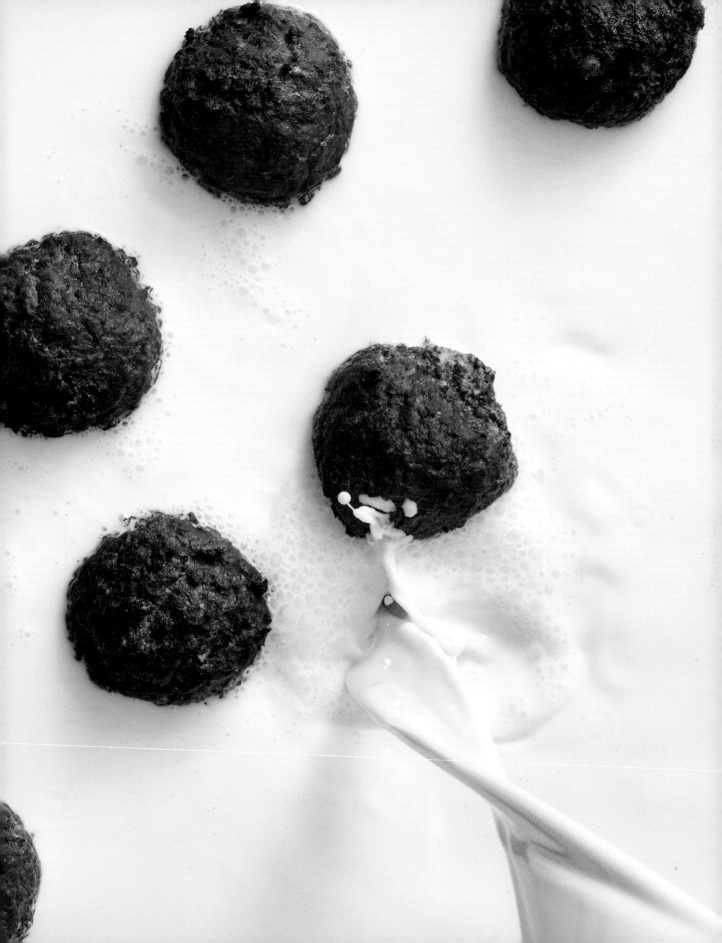

Milk
with
Balls

Week 04

Ingredients

Meatballs

Milk

The liquid we've all grown up with. From the breast to the carton, although I was never allowed to drink straight from the carton. Milk, with a little more substance than you might expect as this treat has lumps. Not the kind you've unexpectedly stumbled upon in your shared-student-fridge. But meat lumps.

More commonly known as meat balls, they've made the jump from the soup bowl to your milk bowl. Or glass if you prefer to not play it safe and drink from a serious choking hazard. The best way to go is to get minced meat and make your own meatballs. Make them as plain or crazy as you want. Some even put feta in them. Fry your balls and heat your milk. Once your balls are done let them cool just a bit and try to dab of the grease before you dunk them in your milk.

Timed best before bed, this hot milk and meatballs beverage, won't only have you sleep tight, it will have you sleep satisfied too. With a milk 'stache. Obviously.

Bananaroni

Ingredients

Spicy Pepperoni

Skewer, not for eating

Bound together by their suggestive shapes and contrasting flavours, these two were made for each other. Bananaroni is their Tinder love child—but unlike other meaning-less one-night stands, this dish is a true keeper. Alternately soft and hard in texture, subtle and outspoken in flavour, it truly has it all.

"Banana again", you ask? Well, it seems bananas are immensely popular amongst moms to be, probably because they're so versatile. They go well with tuna, chocolate, and apparently pepperoni. Plus, they have the added benefit of adding much-needed vitamins to your diet.

Thinly slice the pepperoni, then do the same to the banana. Now stack the two alternately until you've created a bananaroni tower, using a skewer to keep them from falling apart and to make it seem like a party snack. After all, having a baby is a festive occasion.

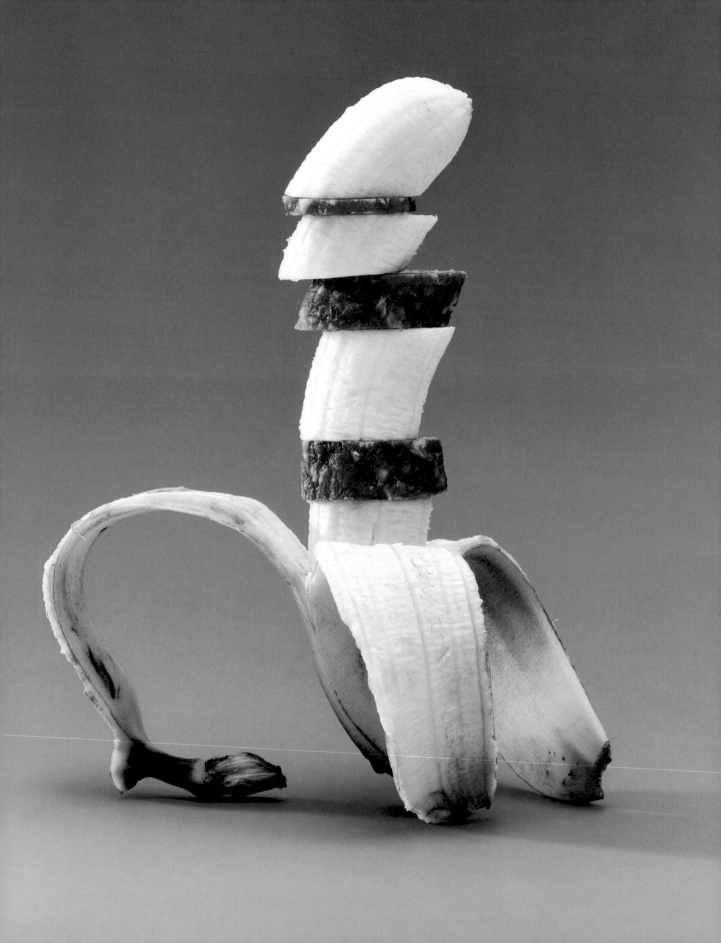

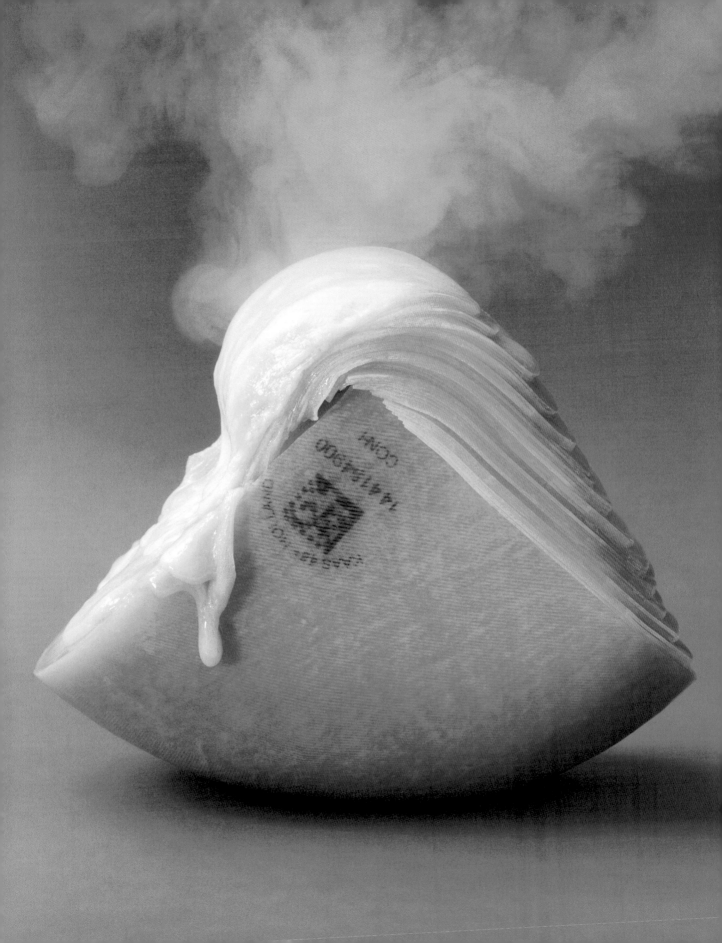

Your baby is now the size of a Lentil or a Lentil-sized crumb of Cheese.

Nuked Gouda

Ingredients

Gouda varying from
0.5 grams to 15 kg

Nuked Cheese or *Nucléaire Fromage* in French is, unsurprising, cheese straight out of the microwave. You don't have to be French to have your heart beat faster over this bland experience, it has excited many nationalities of pregnant women. Visually it's quite the disappointment, but apparently the warm, gooey, and sweaty texture tingles the tastebuds.

All you need to get this thing going is a plate, a microwave, and of course some cheese. Though you're pregnant, and no-one should deny a pregnant lady anything, ever, some cheeses shouldn't be eaten during your pregnancy. Some raw, unpasteurised cheeses could cause listeriosis, a nasty infection that could harm your child or worse. So avoid mould ripened cheeses, unpasteurised cheeses, and uncooked soft blue veined cheeses. Cheeses like Gouda, Edam, Cheddar, Parmesan, Stilton, and even Gruyère are still in the game though.*

*Under no circumstance should the above writings be considered advice or any expert knowledge. ask your GP or health professional what you can or can't consume.

Put the cheese of your craving on a plate, preferably thin slices since this melts the best, and nuke it for about 1 minute at 500W, depending on the amount you've put on the plate. Repeat until the sweaty-goo consistency is to your liking. Bon Apetit?

Week 07

Your baby is now the size of a super small Gherkin or Blueberry.

Pickle juice

Ingredients

Jar of Pickles

Pickles seem to be a pregnancy essential. An ingredient you should have within an arms reach at all times. So stack your pantry with cournichons, bread and butters, genuine dills, and gherkins. Highly multifunctional, they'll always provide a way to satisfy your craving. Even if you're not into pickles. The trick is in the brine.

Diamonds might be a girl's best friend, but pickle juice is a mom-to-be's best friend. In her eyes it's value might very well be worth more than the crown jewels. The juice might not last as long as an actual diamond, but it's odour does. So don't let it drip on your bathrobe when you're gulping it straight out of the jar in the middle of the night.

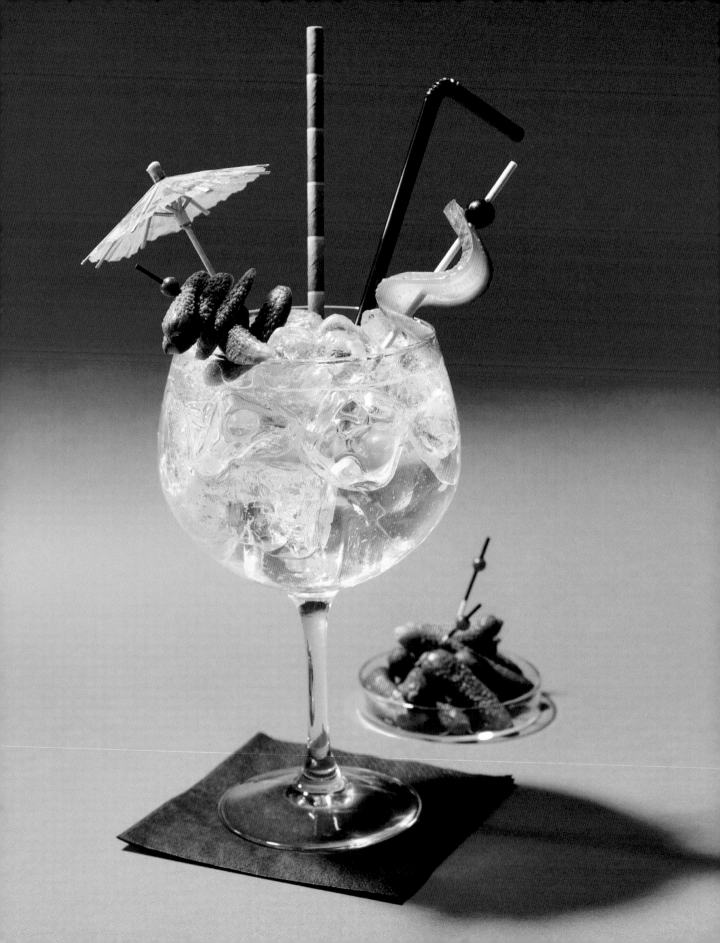

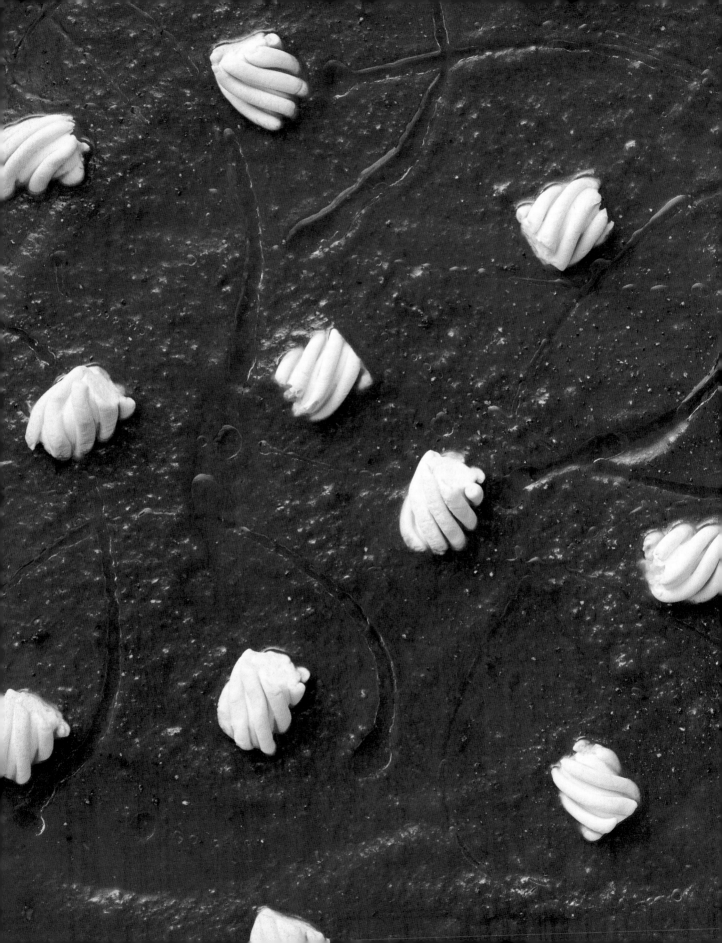

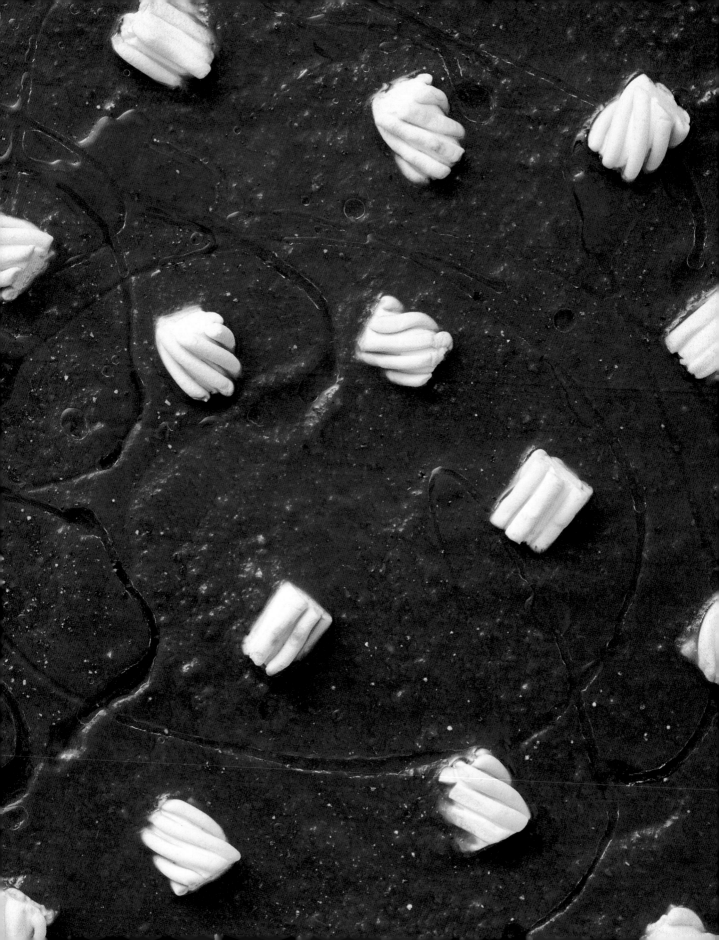

Marsh mallow Gazpacho

Week 08

Ingredients

Canned Tomato Soup

Marshmallows

The one treat we're all too familiar with. Given to us since infancy this ingredient has come full circle. Because, like when you were a toddler, your nerves will be calmed by marshmallows once again. Only this time they will be floating in a Warhol classic. Tomato soup. In fancy food terms: Gazpacho, garnished with some low quality Marshmallows. Whether you're getting Campbell's or an off-brand it doesn't matter as long as it comes straight out of the tin can. Just open it up and dunk your marshmallows in there as if it were hot chocolate.

The attentive readers might notice a pattern in ease. Lots of ladies favour speed above all, which makes sense, really. When you're spending every living second working hard on nurturing your unborn bundle of joy, you deserve a bit of ease. These liquid tomatoes and their soft friends are guaranteed to put your craving to bed.

Your baby is now the size of a tiny Prawn.

Nutty Prawns

Ingredients

100 grams of Shrimp or King Prawns

1 jar of extra chunky Peanut Butter

Like the nutty professor but instead of Eddy, prawns. Cooked prawns covered it peanut butter. Not peanut sauce. A nuance with a big difference I learned firsthand when I made my first 'peanut butter' sandwich as a child.

This actually sounds tasty, although it very much depends on your mise en place. For example, beautifully cooked king prawns served with a smooth spoon of peanut butter on the side with maybe some veggies, could take you back to that nice Thai place where you met your love for the first time. Emptying a box of small shrimp in your extra chunky peanut butter jar is a trip down to Shame-ville, that place residing between guilt and disgust. For you eccentric pregnant eaters however, this could very well be heaven, so add these extra chunks to your peanut butter, give it a good stir, and enjoy your spoon of happiness.

Who cares, go nutty.

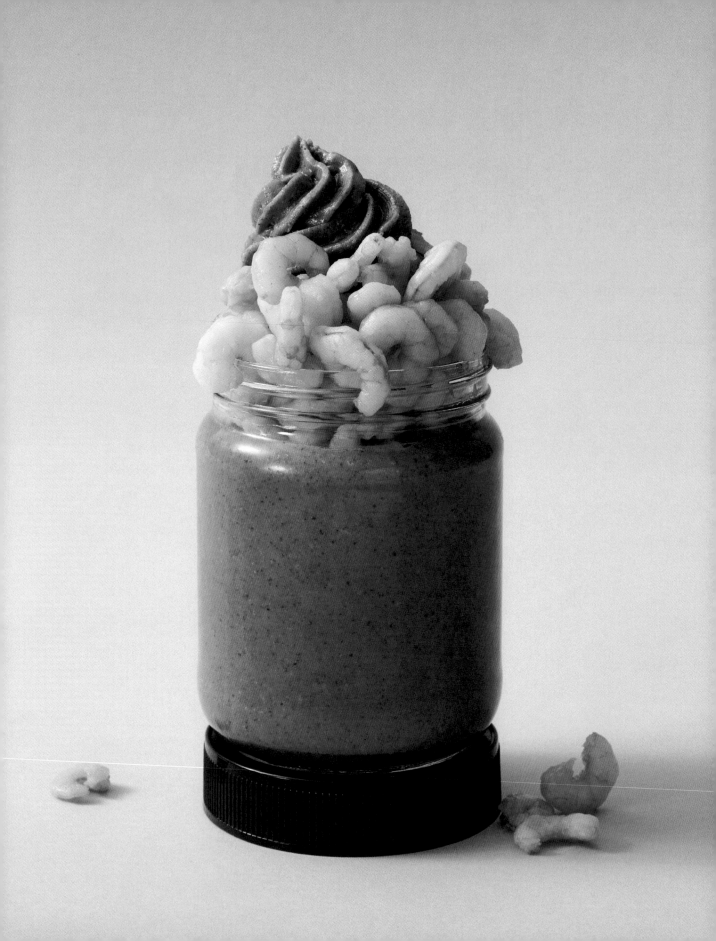

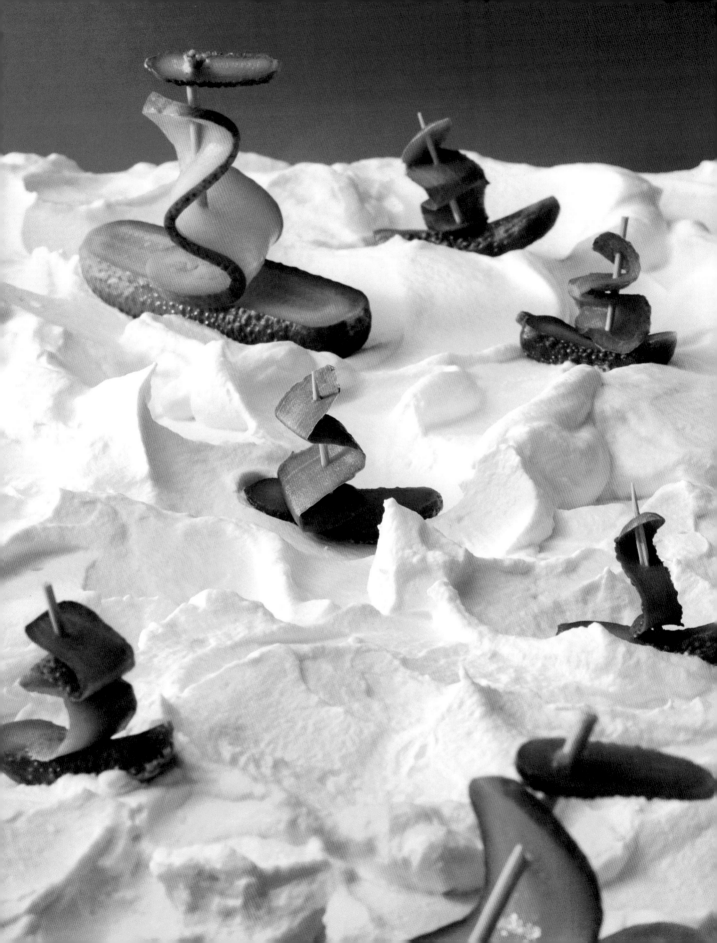

Pickles & Cream

Ingredients

1 jar of uncut Pickles

1 cup of Heavy

Cream

1 pinch of Salt

1 spoon of
Powdered Sugar

A stereotypical treat often featured in pop culture, and rightfully so. The extremes of flavours in this dish appal most of the non-primigravida folks that lay eyes on it, but honestly, this snack has it all. It's flavour is salty, sweet, and sour. It's texture soft, crisp, and crunchy. It's aftertaste? Satisfaction.

Like Rome, there are many ways to whipped pickles—from classy pickle-cream boats or pickles & cream hors d'oeuvre to trashy double dipping or pickle-spraycan-to-the-mouth. In this case we'll go for boats.

Make sure you get the big, un-chopped jumbo ones. Slice them in half; that way you can use them as a carrier for the whipped cream. For the cream you should get heavy cream and whip it manually. Add the sugar and salt, and if you're really feeling adventurous, add vanilla, almond, or anise extract. If the five minutes to whip this up is too much of an effort you can always turn to the spraycans. Though that is highly frowned upon.

Greasy Cucumber

Ingredients

Cucumber

Butter

Chicken

Another great dish you won't have to share, yet it might please the whole family, depending on your execution. The fastest way to satisfaction is some melted butter poured out of over the cucumber, yet this does miss some complexity in flavour and —let's face it—style and will definitely result in some raised eyebrows at home.

The more crafty way of getting to your snack in style, yet remain guilt free, is by covering it in chicken gravy. Not the kind that comes from a packet, but the kind that comes from a real chicken. Whether it is a complete chicken out of the oven or just a leg or wing depends on how much grease you need. My advice would be to prepare a whole chicken and try to get as much grease out of it as you can and then save it in little containers. This enables you to heat up a bit of grease whenever you feel like it. Once your chicken is done, get rid of it. Feed it to the family as if you made it for them with love, we'll know better. When the rest are distracted you can give your full attention to a cucumber with your name on it.

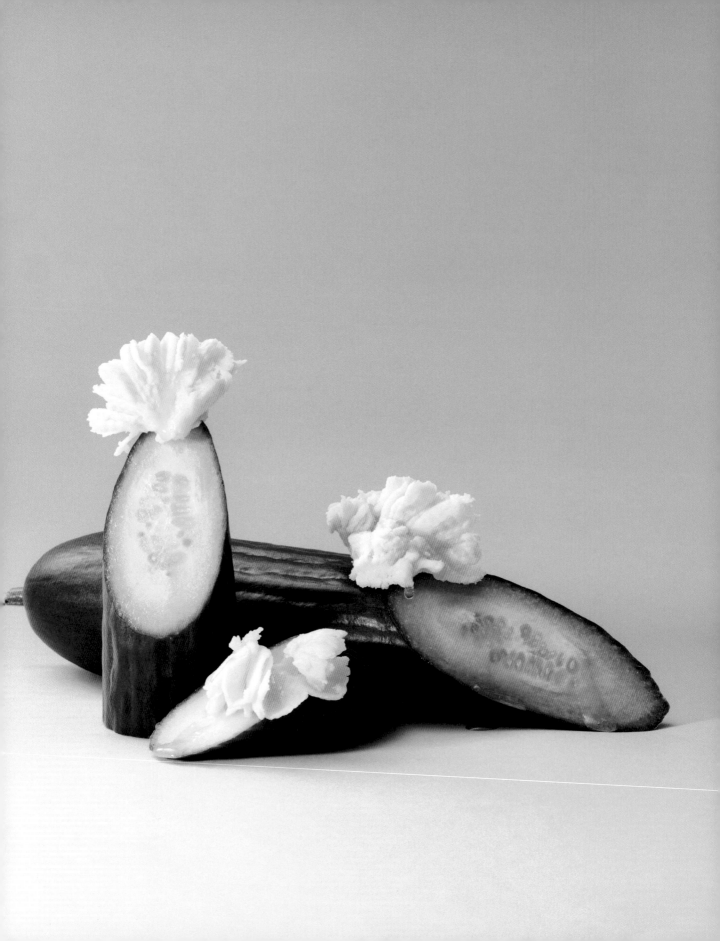

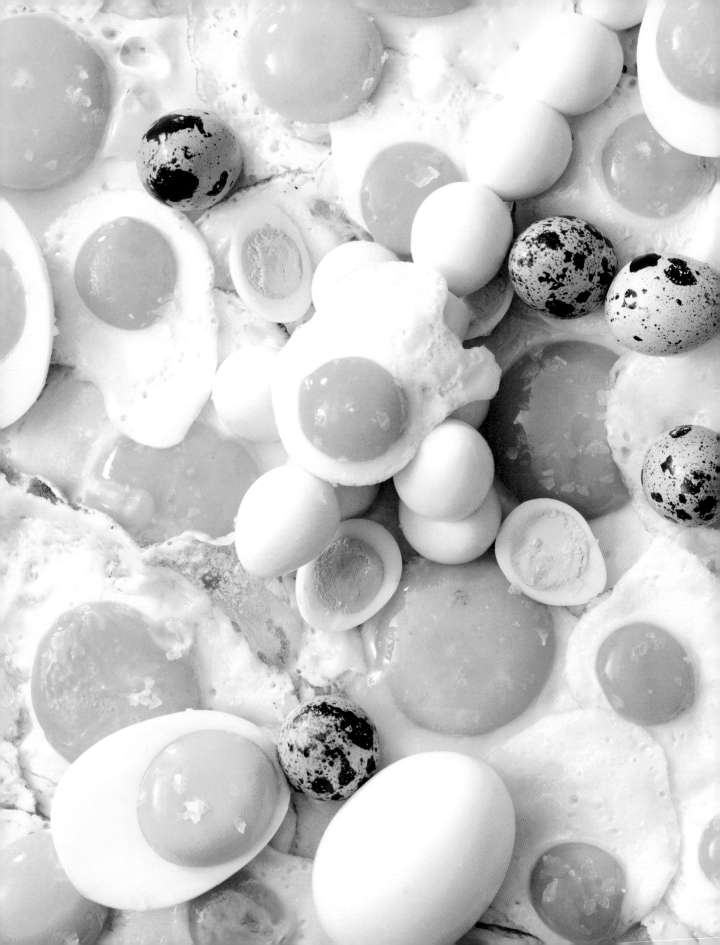

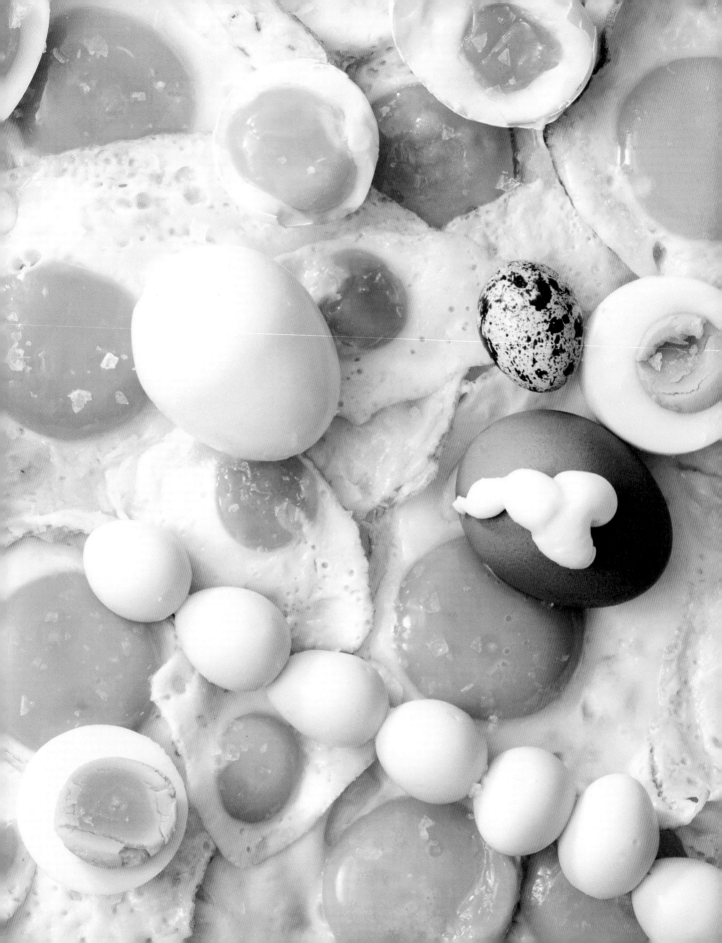

Egg stravagant

Week 12

Your baby is now the size of a Chicken Egg.

Ingredients

Eggs

Eggs

Eggs

Maybe a little toast

Yours might have been fertilised but they're great in many different ways. Eggs that is. Chicken eggs to avoid misunderstandings. Poached, pickled, scrambled, sunny-side up, hard boiled, soft boiled, omelette, Florentine, or Benedict.

Like a lot of things in a pregnancy, it's not an either-or situation but an and, and, and then some more situation. Eggs never come alone, there's a reason you can only buy them by the six, ten, or a dozen. That reason is you. You can't O.D. on eggs, but your arteries won't like it in the long run. So whenever you indulge in this eggstravagant spread enjoy it, just don't repeat it every day. With this recipe life will be served sunny side up.

Week 13

Your baby is now the size of a Peach. Also great with Nutella.

Nutella fingers

Ingredients

180 grams Nutella jar, or

200 grams Nutella jar, or

400 grams Nutella jar, or

750 grams Nutella jar, or

1000 grams Nutella jar, or

All of the above

Remember Joey from "Friends"? He came up with the perfect snack for Thanksgiving: peanut butter-fingers. A simple idea, and as most simple ideas go they often turn out to be the best ones. Well, this is basically the same thing but with Nutella. With a global production of about 350 million kilos a year, we can hardly call Nutella a pregnancy craving exclusive. However, most non-pregnant people can withstand the urge to stick their fingers in a Nutella jar. The question is, can you?

Although simple, it's a dish that still offers some options. Mainly volume options. Will you get the humble 180 grams jar or the colossal 3kg? The latter will probably end in Nutella fists though, but if the hand fits...

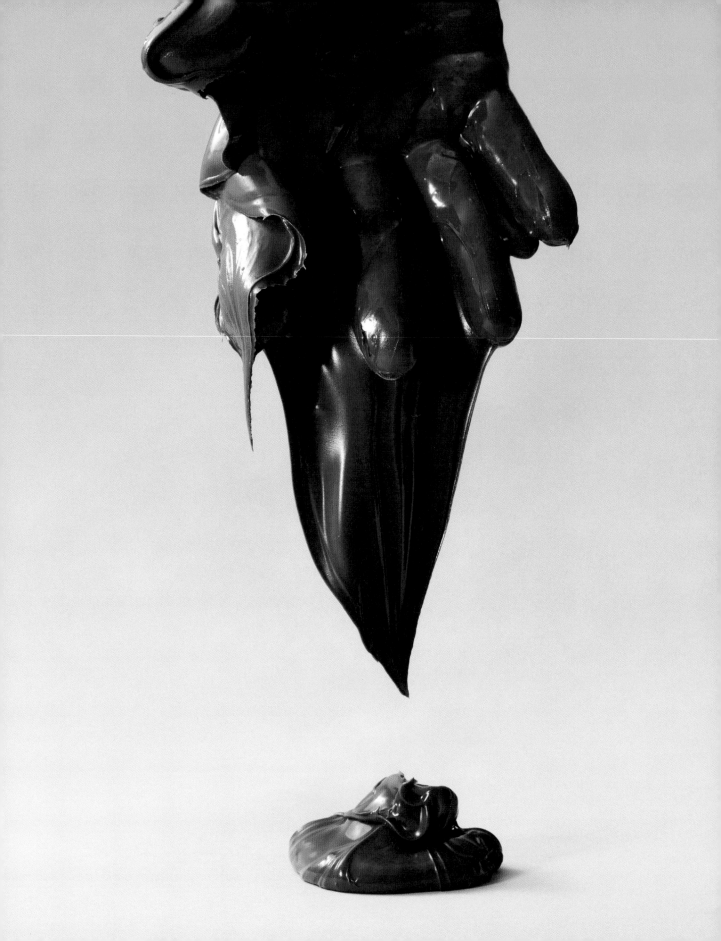

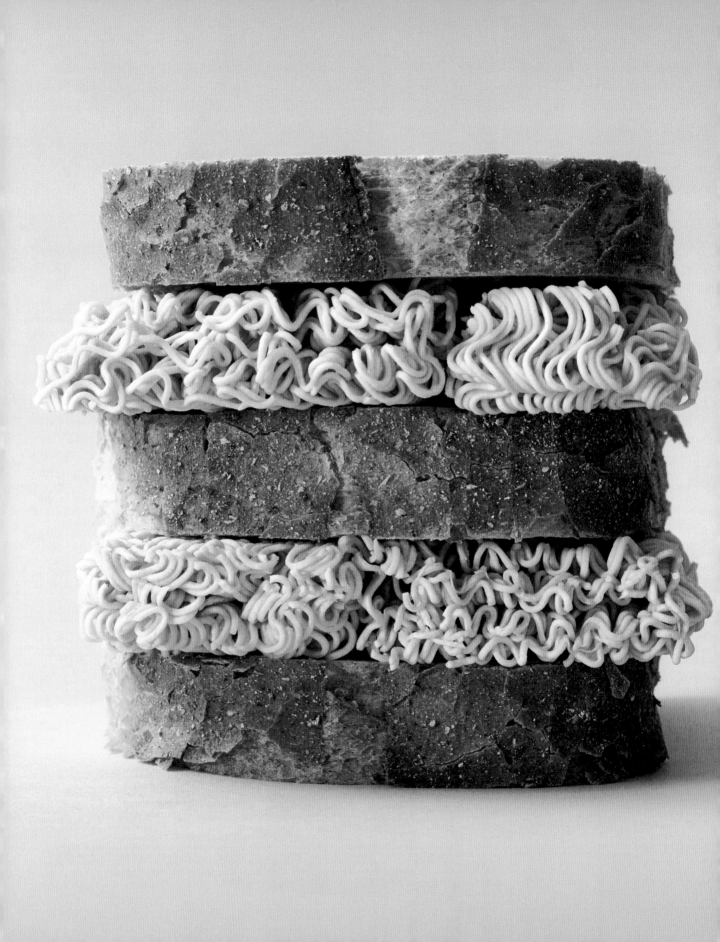

Instant Sandwich

Ingredients

Instant Pot Noodles

Two slices of
Whole Wheat Bread

Technically this counts as an asian fusion dish, but this recipe is far from a gastronomic pinnacle. In fact, many chefs would consider it the exact opposite. Admittedly, it's a very creative recipe with lots and lots of texture, but don't expect a Michelin star for putting this bad boy together.

This perfect crunchy breakfast sandwich is intended to soothe the urges for texture and crunchy mouthfeel. Although a toaster can add a significant crunch to your breakfast, it stands no chance against these noodles. Instant pot noodles. Uncooked and without the pot. The purist would just stack the brick of dried noodles between two slices of bread. However, if you're feeling adventurous, you could also crumble the noodles and sprinkle it through a sandwich of your choice. Just make sure you use whole wheat bread, you need nutrition after all. If, besides crunch, you're also looking for flavour with some texture, add the herbs, garlic, and chili oil from the herb-packet. Now, crush that sub as if you were captain crunch. Instant satisfaction.

Potato Palooza

Ingredients

A substantial amount
of Potatoes

Even when you're not pregnant there is never such a thing as too many potatoes. There are about 4,000 species of different kinds of potatoes out there all waiting to be conquered by you. From the Adirondack Blue, Purple Peruvian, or Bonotte to the Doré and Eigenheimer they all deserve a place on your plate.

Get them cooked, fried, baked, barbecued, ovened, hasselbacked, rose-married, or mashed. Make a gratin, soup, salad, chips, hash browns, latkes, tator tots, patattas bravas, or potato gnocchi. This will be the potato plate of plates. As you can have them all. And you will have them all. But this much goodness comes at a price. The price of imagination. Which is great in the kitchen, but it might seriously put a dent in your creditcard bill if you're overly creative. A Bonotte potato comes at a price of €500 per kilo so pick your spuds carefully.

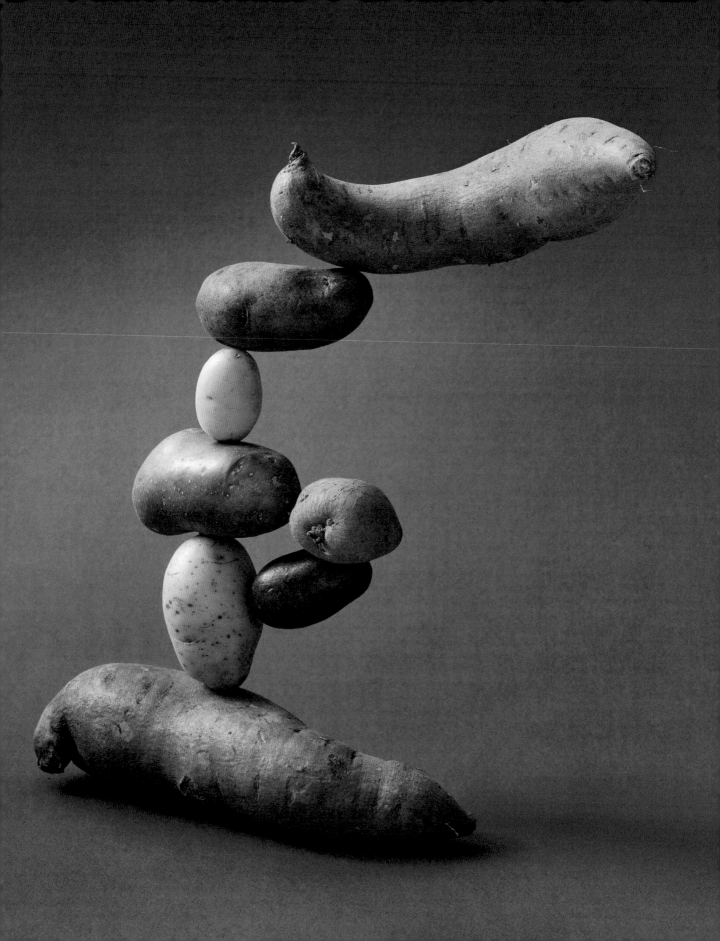

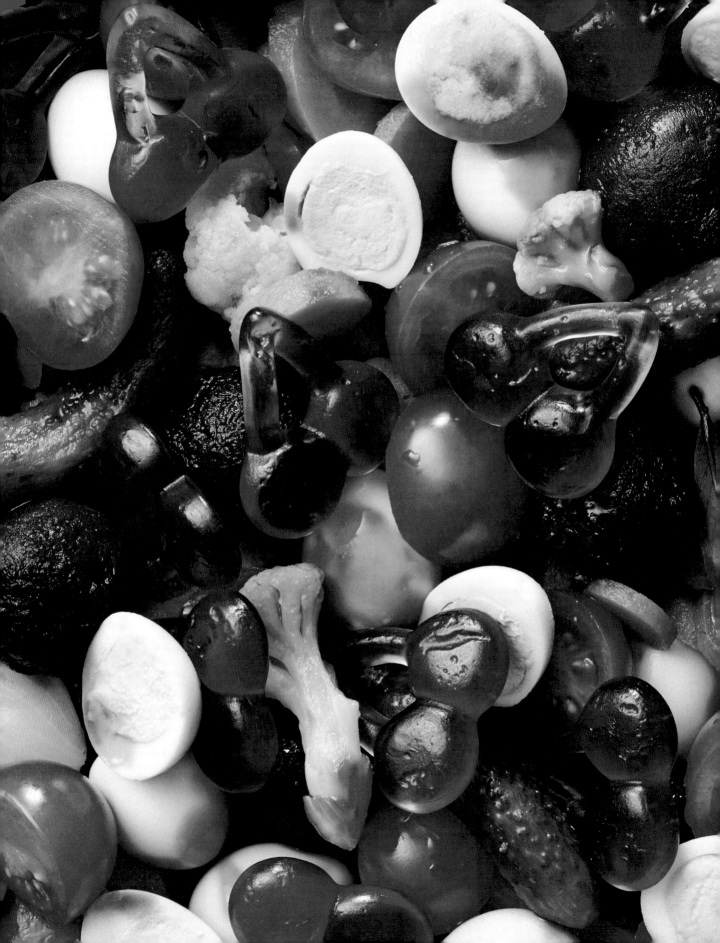

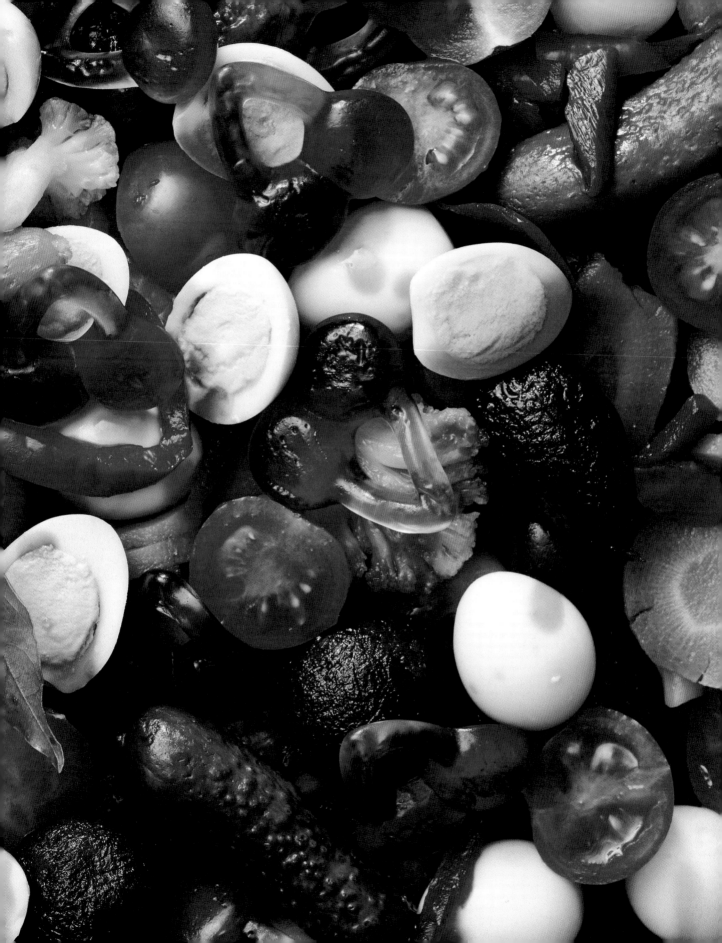

.Pickled
insomnia

Week 16

Your baby is now as big as an 11.5 cm sized Beet. Also great to pickle.

Ingredients

Salt

Sugar

Vinegar

Water

Pick your ingredient

Pair your compulsive craving with some compulsive action, and hit two birds with one pickle, by pickling everything. Now, you not only get to eat your weird craving at god-knows-what-hour, you also get to make it. Not an unwelcome surprise as it will give you something to do while battling your first trimester insomnia.

Instead of lying in bed wide awake, pickling stuff can be a great way to distract your mind from those sleep depriving thoughts, and will make you some great midday snacks. Pickle yourself some onions, carrots, cauliflower, cherries, gherkins, beetroot, asparagus, peppers, tomatoes, eggplant, eggs, asian pears, or plums. You name it and you can probably pickle it.

Mix a cup of water with a cup of vinegar of choice, like white, rice, or apple, and add two tablespoons of pickling salt and one tablespoon of granulated sugar. Boil it over high heat until the salt and sugar are dissolved. Pack a jar full of your ingredient of choice and poor the brine in until one centimeter from the top.

This snack is great to be made in the middle of the night, just don't eat it. This will only fuel your insomnia and that will leave you in a whole other kind of pickle.

Your baby is now the size of an Onion. A big one, not a small one.

Random Trifle

Ingredients

Roasted Almonds

Pickeld Onions

Cottage Cheese

By random, I mean almond-and-pickled-onion-cottage-cheese-triffle random. How? I can't even... How does anyone come up with this random selection of ingredients? The craving force must have been strong in the one that chowed this one down. I'm guessing the almonds give the cottage cheese a nice crunch? Notice that I wrote "guessing". I was raised in a, tryeverything,-you-don't-know-if-you-like-it,-if-you-haven't-eaten-it' kind of way, but this concoction would even have my dad go straight for his pudding.

But someone, somewhere, got excited by this peculiar selection of ingredients, so if it floats your boat have at it. Start with a layer of almonds in the bottom of your bowl. Make sure the entire bottom is covered and cover it in cottage cheese. Then make a layer of pickled onions. Again make sure it completely covers the other layer before you cover it in cottage cheese again. Make another layer of almonds and cover it in cottage cheese until it's nice and flat. Put one onion and almond on top if you feel culinary. There you have it. A trifle that will haunt my dad in his dreams. Eat tight.

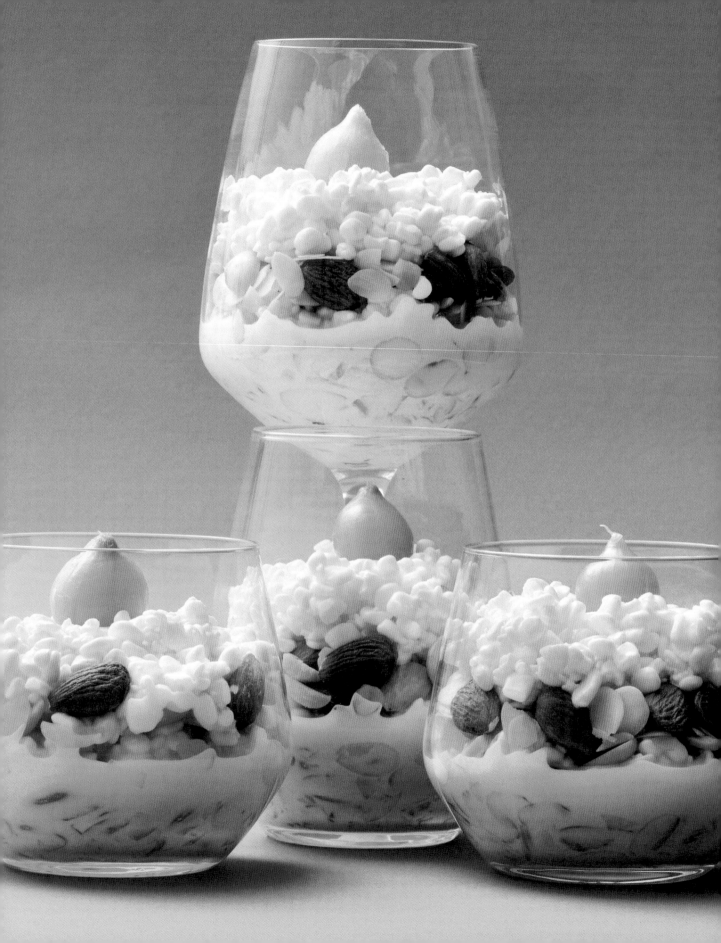

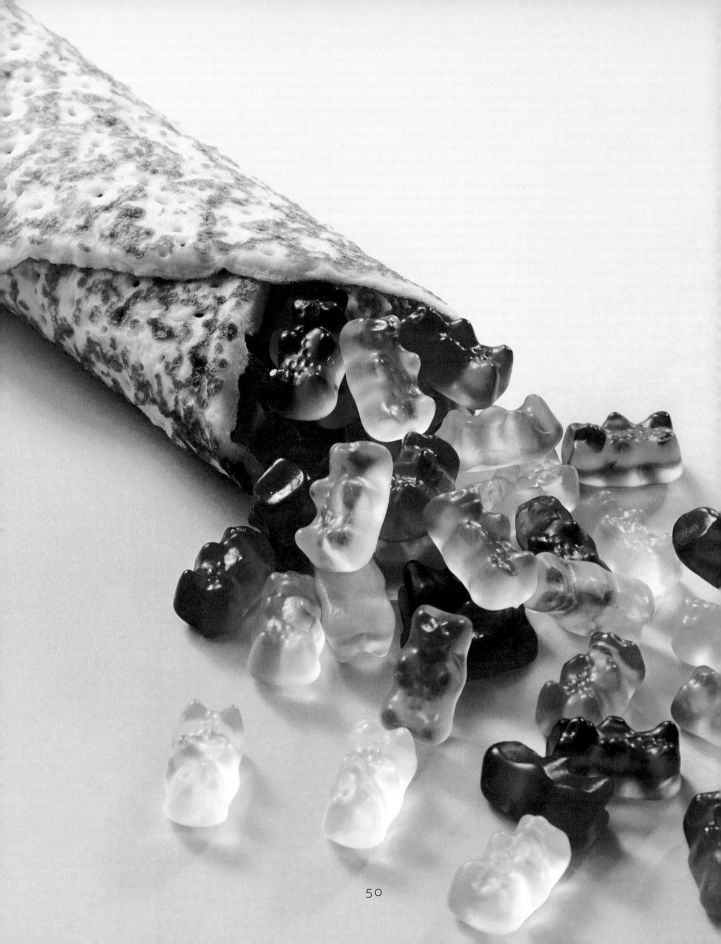

Gummy-Bear Crêpe

Ingredients

250 g Flour

2 Eggs

500 ml Milk

A little bit of Cinnamon

Gummy Bears

If Peter Pan had written a cookbook, this gummy bear-infused crêpe suzette recipe would be on the front cover. It lets you connect with the kid inside of you—I mean your inner kid, not the one connected to your umbilical cord. Bright, colourful gummy bears melted or sprinkled on your crêpe sounds like an odd choice, but some swear by it.

Put the flour, eggs, and milk in a bowl and whisk them smooth—a mixer will help you to get a fluffy batter. Add a teaspoon of cinnamon for flavour. Now pour one big full soupspoon into a pan and let it settle for a second before dropping the gummy bears on top. Make sure the top is still wet and the bottom dry. If you're OCD as well as pregnant, add only red bears. Or orange. Or green, for peace of mind. If you love surprises, hide the bears in your pancake by covering them in some more batter. Flip the pancake over and make sure it's cooked through.

If this pregnancy isn't your first rodeo, make sure your other kids aren't around, or you'll be sharing.

Cheesy Freezy Peas

Ingredients

Small to medium sized
Green Peas

Cottage Cheese

Some child-bearing ladies find great cravings to be like revenge, a meal best served cold. In this case ice-cold at a whopping -18°C. Frozen peas with cottage cheese—a dish that is one spelt cracker and eighteen degrees away from being the new health-hyped-food trend.

First, you need to make sure you get regular green peas, not chickpeas or any other bigger kind of pea. You want to freak out on it, not choke on it. In this case, smaller is better. You can make a whole culinary adventure out of this in presentation. Peas on a bed of cottage cheese, the other way around, or how most of you probably prefer it, in the cottage cheese container. The faster it's ready, the better. So just dump a hand full of peas in your cottage cheese, grab a fork, and go nuts. Or actually, peas.

For the people around the person eating it, beware: this craving is a good indicator of a revengeful character, or a really healthy person. In either case, don't step on their toes, especially not in their condition.

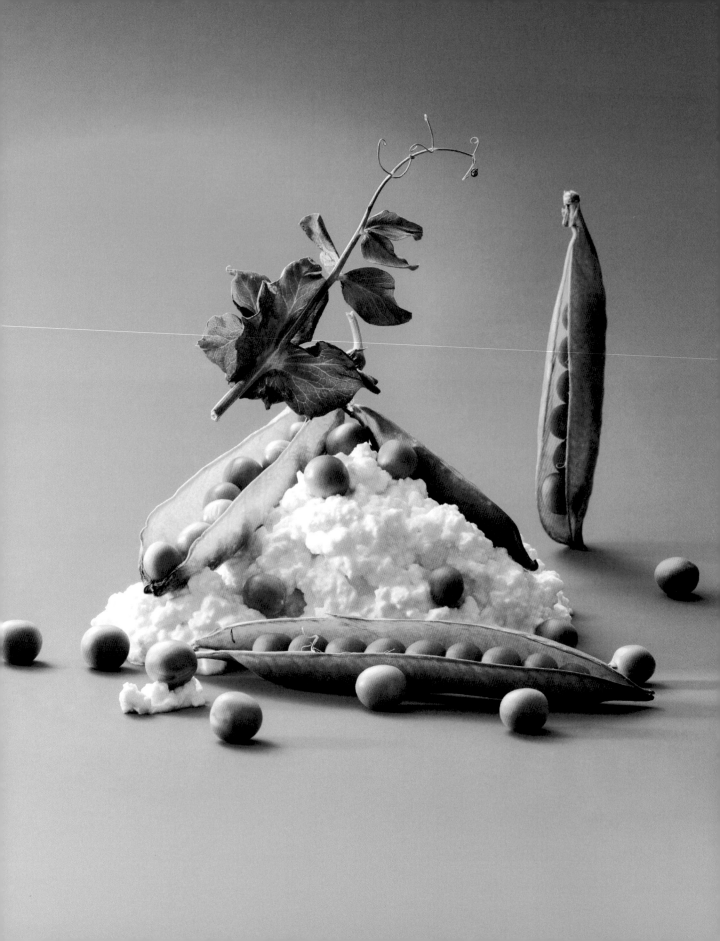

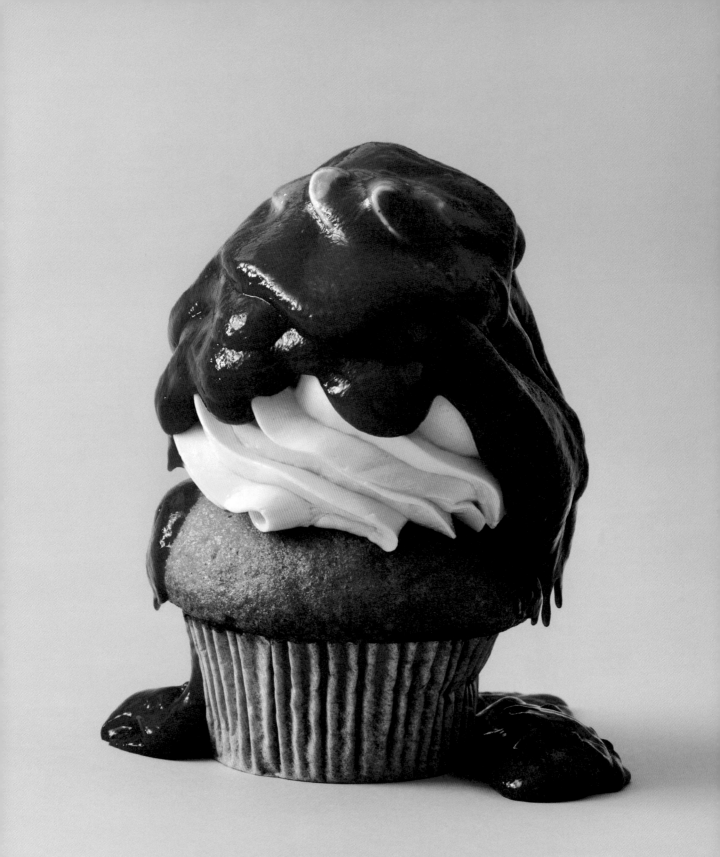

Everything Ketchup

Ingredients

The biggest bottle
of Heinz Ketchup
you can find

Having always played second fiddle in the realm of food, it is time to get it off the sideline of life and give it the rightful place it deserves. Main course, primo piatto, the *pièce de résistance*. Ketchup. The beauty of this recipe is that you can and should use it on any type of food of your craving. You can make it as cheap and fast or expensive or expansive as you'd like. The brand of choice? Heinz. No, this is not product placement, it's objective product preference. Because, as Malcolm Gladwell* once stated in The New Yorker, Heinz uniquely hits on all five tastes: sweet, sour, salty, bitter, and umami.

Spread this tomato goodness on caviar, cantaloupes, cup cakes, or cookies. Smother your mother's potatoes, peas, pear, papayas, or paprikas in it. If you're still in the cheese phase, grab some parmesan, gouda, or edam and drown it in ketchup. Though, with it being Heinz, all it takes is a little patience. Then again, good things come to those who wait.

*Malcolm Gladwell, August 29, 2004. *The Ketchup Conundrum*, The New Yorker.

Tunana

Ingredients

Any canned John
West Tuna or
Catfood (if cat)

Banana

Bowl

Depending on the size of your wallet you can go with fresh tuna steak, or you can step in our simpleton footsteps and get yourself some canned tuna. Not the cat food, although it's packaged similarly. You're gonna have a bad time with cat food. Unless you're a feline with opposable thumbs. Though, if that was the case, you'd probably have enslaved all of mankind and made them poop in a litterbox.

Tuna is only fifty percent of this disturbing dish. The other half? Banana. Empty the whole tuna can in a bowl and stir it with some salt and pepper. Now it's time to go crazy, peel a banana and slice it up in the bowl. I know you can't wait to get your claws in this one but wait just a minute. Stir the whole lot again and get the juices of the tuna soaked into the banana. Eat it with a fork, or if you are the supreme feline leader, have it fed to you.

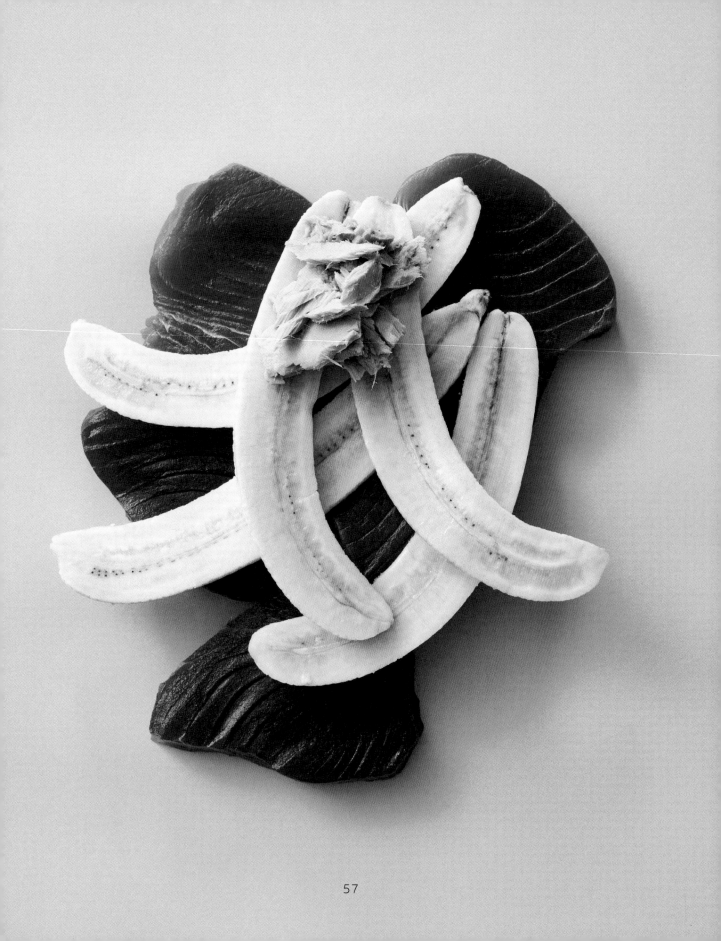

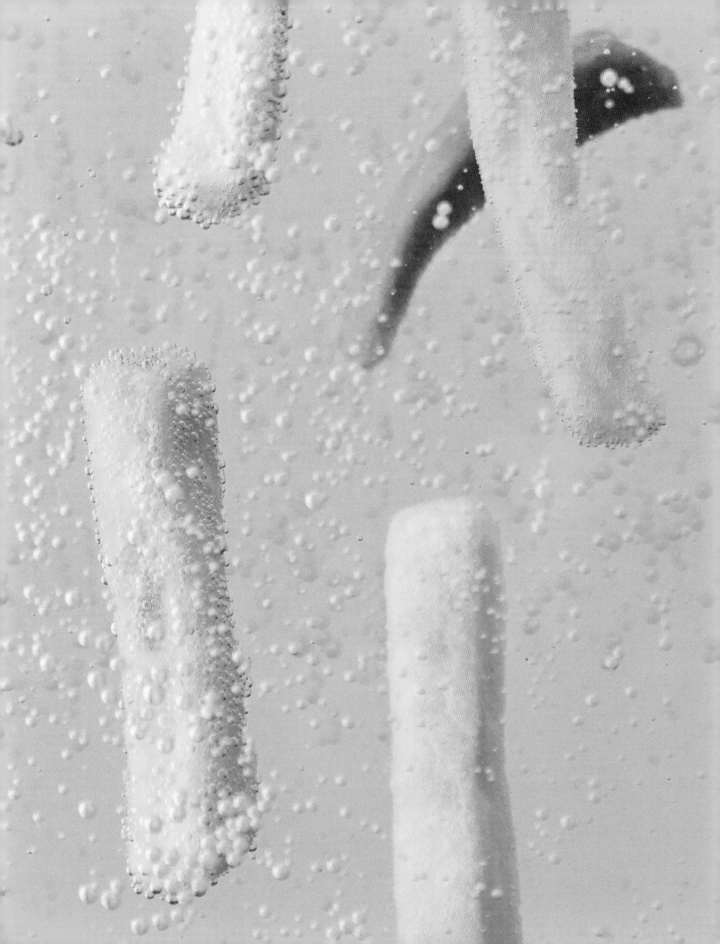

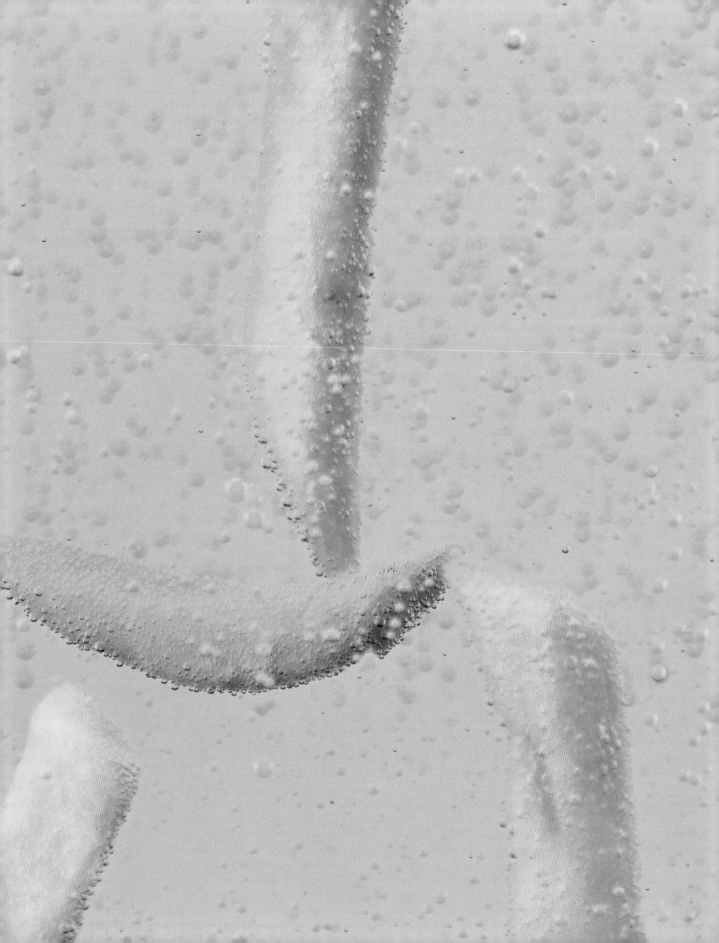

French
Fry
Ginger
Beer

Week 22

Your baby is now as tall as a Carrot or a really long French Fry.

Ingredients

Ginger Beer

French Fries

Neither shake nor solid food, this is the perfect hybrid for when you don't know what you want, a common problem when you're pregnant. Liquid with a bite, sort off. For this snack, instead of ice cubes in your drink, you'll have fries. French fries, or if you feel adventurous, Belgian.

I can't put my finger on what makes this snack work so well, but I can attest that it slips down easily, and I'm a non-pregnant male. Though I do have a thing for fries, so it might not be for everyone.

Fill a glass with French fries, completely stuff it to the top, then drown it in ginger beer. Don't let it settle too long as the fries will become soggy, unless soggy fries are your thing.

Week 23

Your baby is now as big as a 26 to 30 cm stack of Sour Cream containers.

Sour cream *to go*

Ingredients

Sour Cream

Sour Cream

Sour Cream

Sour Cream

Sour Cream

Sour Cream

Sometimes you just don't have the time to prepare an extensive meal and you just need a quick fix, like the Pocket Honey recipe you'll find nine pages from here, for example. Although it has a similar ease to it, you don't want to keep this one in your pocket, for obvious reasons. It is more a straight out of the fridge kind of thing. The longer sour cream stays out of the fridge the dodgier it gets. So empty it in one go. Take a big spoon, tear of the lidd and just let your emotional eater unleash itself.

Unlike cheese there's no issue with eating sour cream in the context of your baby. In the context of your baby fat however, there is. Sour cream is BFF with your BBF and, depending on whether you want to embrace it or shake it, you might want to keep track of the excess. Your craving will eventually leave you, your BBF however is here to stay.

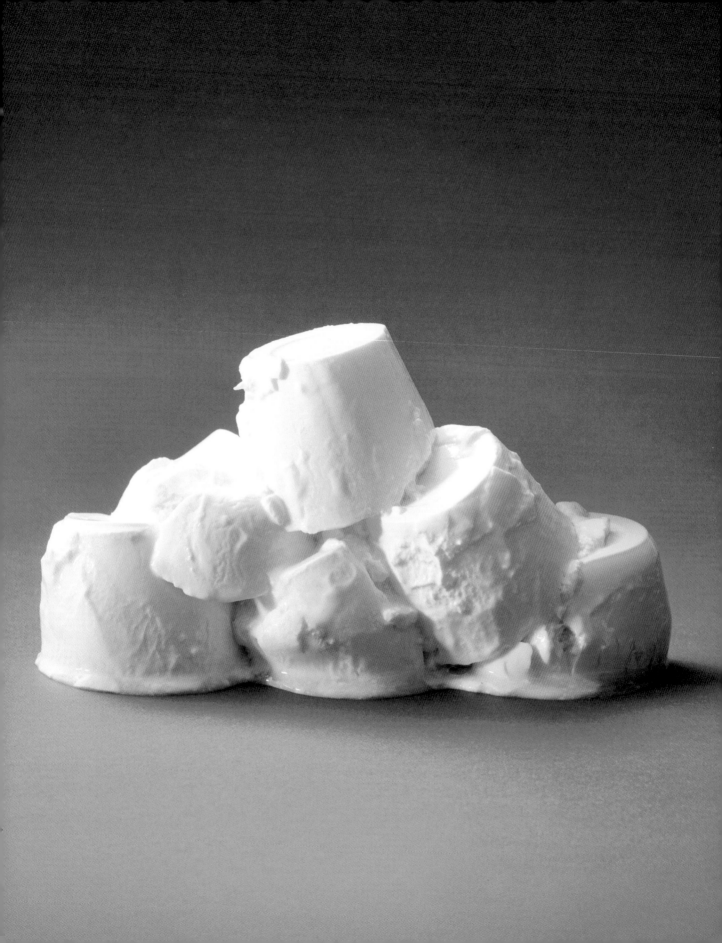

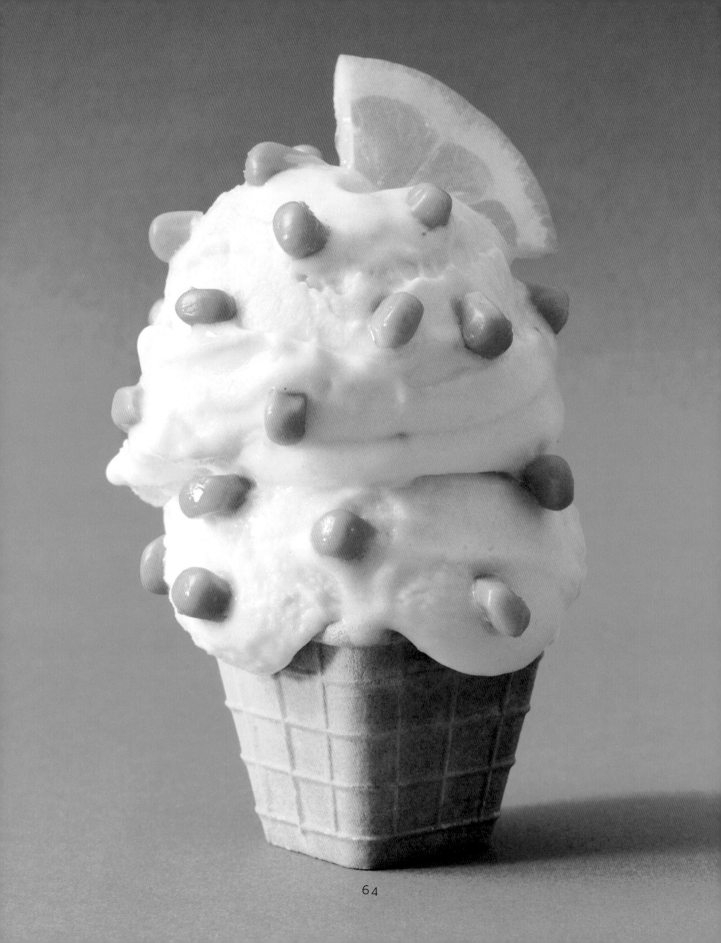

Yellow Snow

Ingredients

Canned Corn

Lemon Ice Cream

Being the rebel you are you can finally go against the age-old rule of not eating the yellow snow. Though it's solid advice, not all yellow snow is not for eating. The snow we talk about is not the kind your drunken partner, immature dad, or golden retriever makes. This one is chunky and slightly more appealing since it's made of canned corn and lemon ice cream.

Like many dishes in this book you can dress this one up or down, depending on your craving. Keep it simple and open a tin of corn and add as many scoops of lemon ice cream in there as fits. Just stuff it in there. Just don't lick it straight out. The razor-sharp edge of the can, can make the yellow snow turn red—which benefits no one—so use protection and get in there with a spoon.

Go fancy and get your favourite handcrafted ceramic bowl and carefully place a perfect scoop of lemon ice cream in there and sprinkle it with corn kernels. Or go classic, get some ice-cream cones, place your scoops on top, and decorate it with corn kernels as if it's disco dip. Do it. Eat the yellow snow.

A fistful of Cheese

Ingredients

Mozarella

Washed hands

This has nothing to do with Clint Eastwood duelling cowboys. Cows, however, do play a part in this very basic bite. Mozzarella straight out of your hand. No plate, no napkin, nom nom nom. It's the sheer basicness of this tremendously satisfying snack that makes it such a succes. That it's one of the few cheeses you're allowed to eat coming months plays a small part in it too. But this cheesy medal has a dark side, too. Not like Vader but that it is fifty-five percent fat. Fifty-five. Percent. A pretty steep number, but I know your craving isn't intimidated by this one single bit. It eats numbers like that for breakfast. And lunch. Maybe even as an afternoon snack with some tea. If the frequency rises to such levels, you need to find your fix in one of the other tasty titles I have listed before and after this recipe. Because there's no way you can disguise fifty-five percent fat three times a day as baby fat. So stuff responsibly.

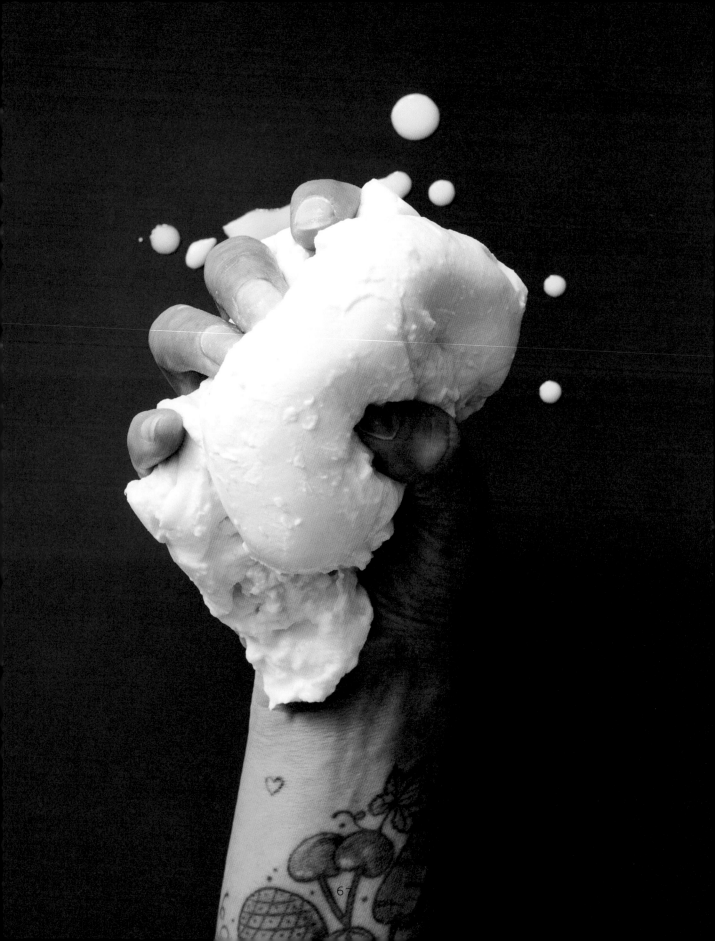

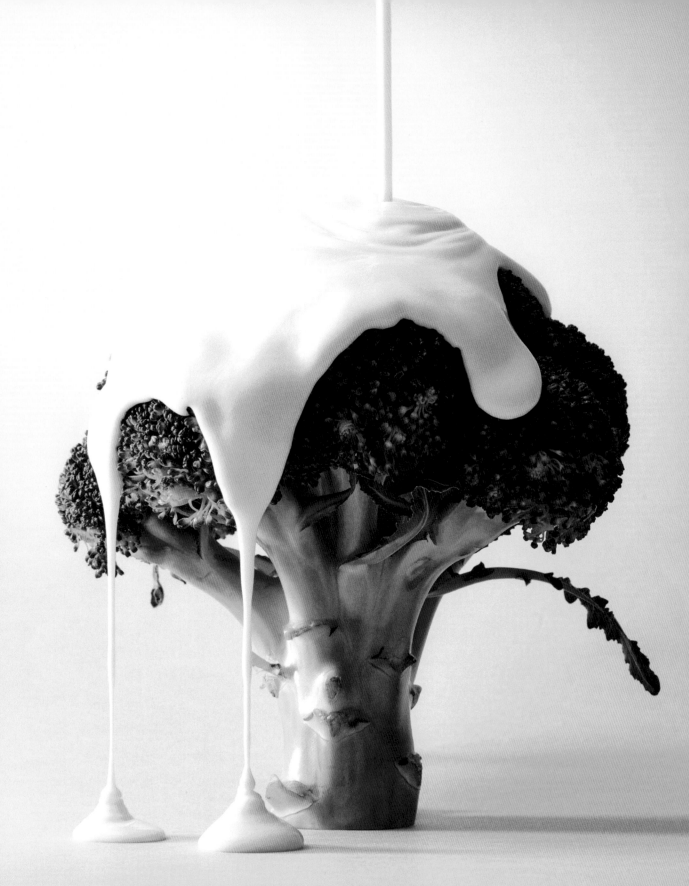

Broghurt

Ingredients

One Brocoli

Full Yoghurt

Peper and Salt

Though the title sounds like it came from some obscure frat-boy vocabulary, this dish has nothing to do with the satisfaction of man. However, it has everything to do with the satisfaction of women. Pregnant women. Think yoghurt. The kind you have with granola. Thick, full yoghurt with some surprises beneath the surface. A surprise ruined by the poor title. Brocoli. Fresh Brocoli. Greens in my maidenly, white, unblemished Yoghurt, you ask? Well, know that we're not talking that cooked-to-death excuse of a vegetable your mom and dad used to ruin Sunday evenings with.

We're talking crisp, crunchy, vivid green Brocoli that you can pick up at your basic Supermarket or organic grower if you want. If your feet are killing you or if you're just lazy, frozen Brocoli will be fine too, but defrost it first. We don't judge.

Cut it up in nice little pieces of an inch or two and blanché it in a pot of boiling water, without the lid on, for about two to three minutes with some pepper and salt. After which you let it rest in a bowl of cold water. We don't want it sweating in our yoghurt. Once cooled down, drown as much Brocoli as you like in your yoghurt.

Life is bro.

Kimchi

Ingredients

Korean supermarket
Kimchi - or

Cabbage

Carrot

Daikon

Garlic

Ginger

Chili Powder

Cayenne Powder

Bean Paste

Oyster/Fish Sauce

A delicacy to Koreans and basically any Korean cuisine aficionado. These fermented vegetables are quite present in taste, hence it sparks such interest amongst pregnant women. It comes in all shapes and sizes but is a bit harder to come by than your average recipe. You can get it at any Korean supermarket, but depending on where you live, you might need to make it yourself. And that takes preparation and patience.

All right, here we go. Take some Chineses cabbage like pak choi or daikon, chop it to the size of your liking and put it in a bowl with four cups of water and four tablespoons of salt. Make sure everything is soaked in the water, otherwise add more water and salt in the same proportion. Let it set for a couple of hours, or overnight. While waiting make a paste of minced garlic, ginger, chili powder, cayenne powder, bean paste, and oyster- or fish sauce. Take the cabbage out of the water and taste it. It should be lightly salty. If it's too salty rinse it down. Mix the cabbage, daikon, and carrot with the paste thoroughly and stuff it in glass jars, like maison jars. Now the waiting game begins. The longer you wait the better it gets. About a week or two you should already be able to eat it, but if you have a strong mind it's best to wait a month.

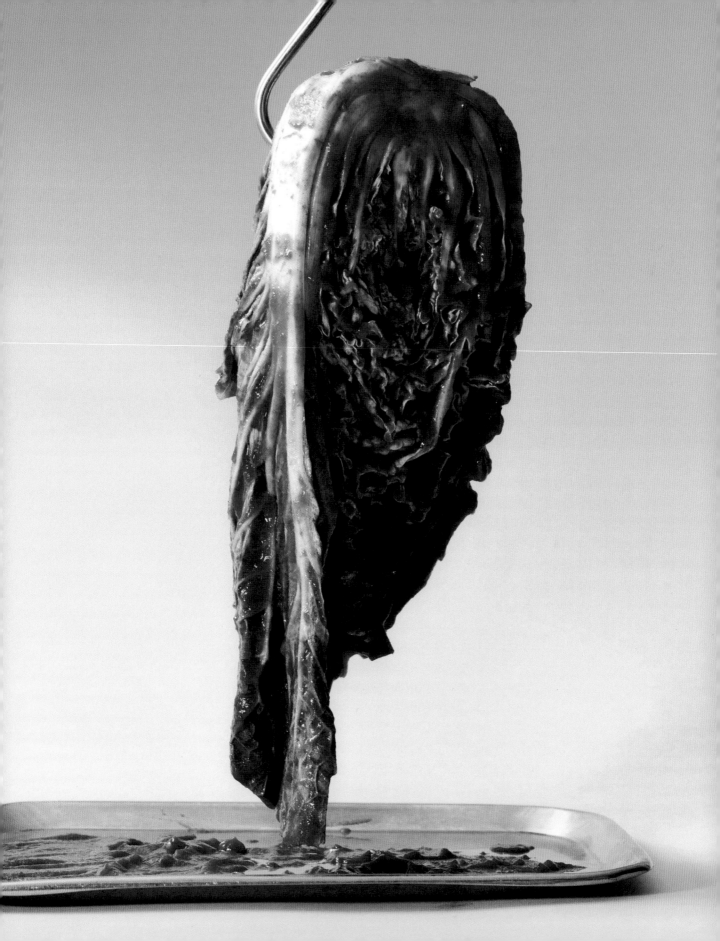

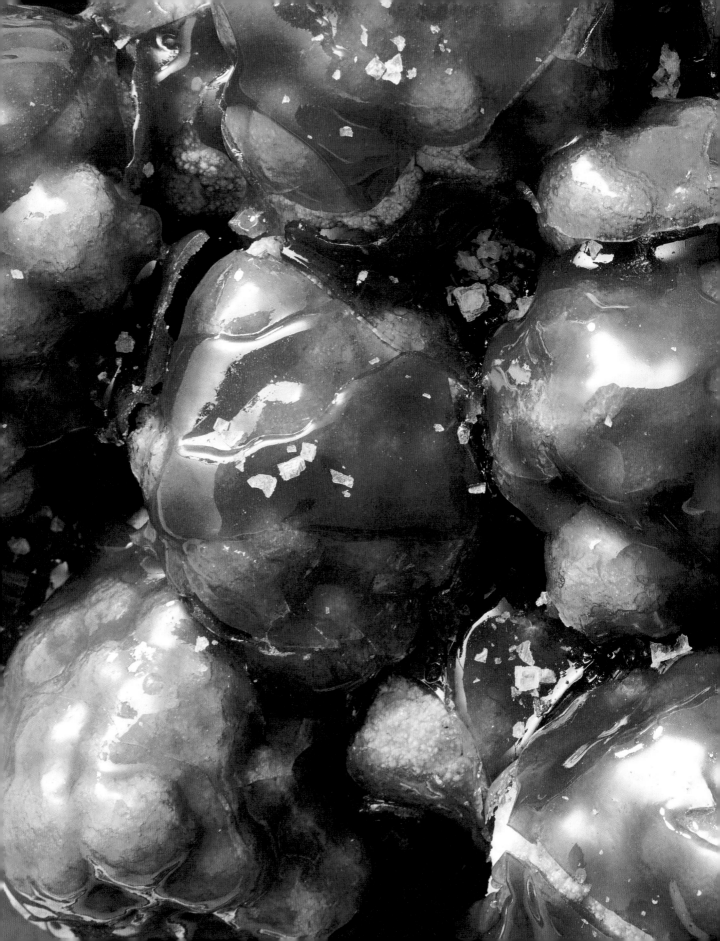

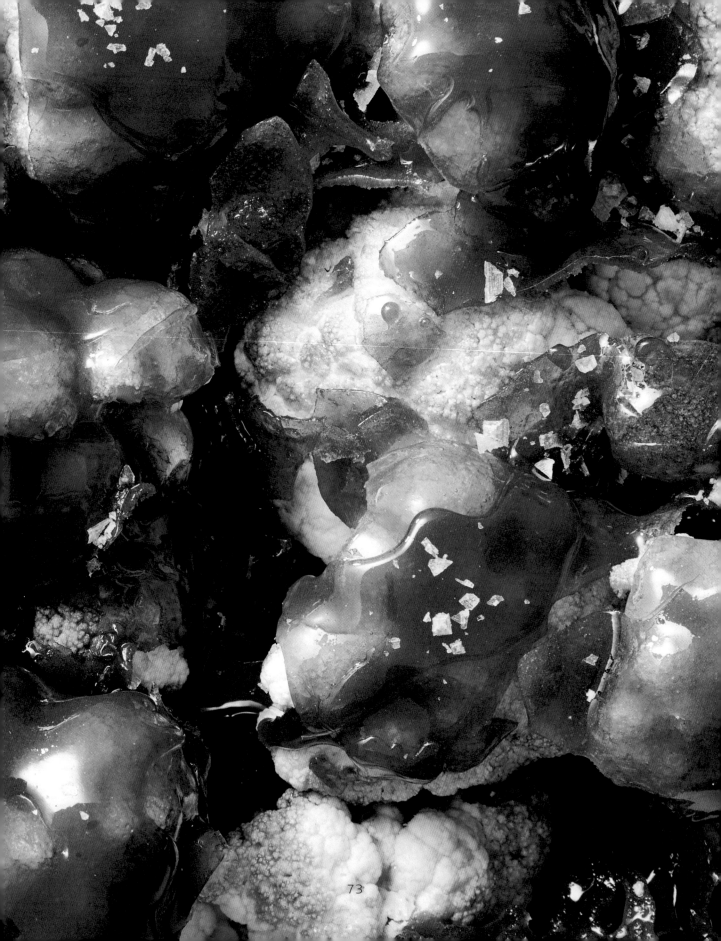

cc

Week 28

Ingredients

Cauliflower

Salted Caramel

Some of you might already be OOO (Out Of Office) for a while, enjoying your maternity leave. And although this title reminds you of the endless stressed out e-mail bombardments your colleague Daryll used to send, it has very little to do with it. CC is just a poorly composed abbreviation of a recipe involving Caramel and Cauliflower. Blanched cauliflower. Because the whole point of this recipe is texture. The feeling of chewing through something that has a bit of crunch, some resistance, something that makes you work for it and has a clear presence in your mouth. So under no circumstance should you aim to boil it.

Cut and wash the cauliflower and boil it in a pot of water for three minutes after which you submerge it in an ice bath. Once it's cold to the touch you can take it out. While it is cooling melt some sugar, add some butter and cream and poor it out over the cauliflower until it sets. There you go. Chewy, crispy caramel cauliflower. C-C-C-C.

Week 29

Your baby is now the size of a Kabocha Squash or a giant Meatball.

Ovalries

Ingredients

Round edible stuff

Sometimes cravings don't limit themselves to taste buds. Some pregnant women are transformed overnight from law-abiding citizens into rampant kleptomaniacs. Others are attracted to particular shapes rather than flavours, which is what this recipe is all about: circles and ovals. Eating them, not stealing them.

Use anything round or oval that you can stuff your face with. Think cheese balls, carrot balls, chocolate balls, meatballs, potato balls, Brussels sprouts, peas, oranges, tangerines, donuts or donut holes. The mouthfeel is the main purpose here, so don't gobble down 15 chocolate balls all at once. Eating them one by one is what truly gets this craving rolling.

Combine the different foods to create pairings of flavour and texture. Eat from small to big, or the other way around. Juggle them in any way you deem fit.

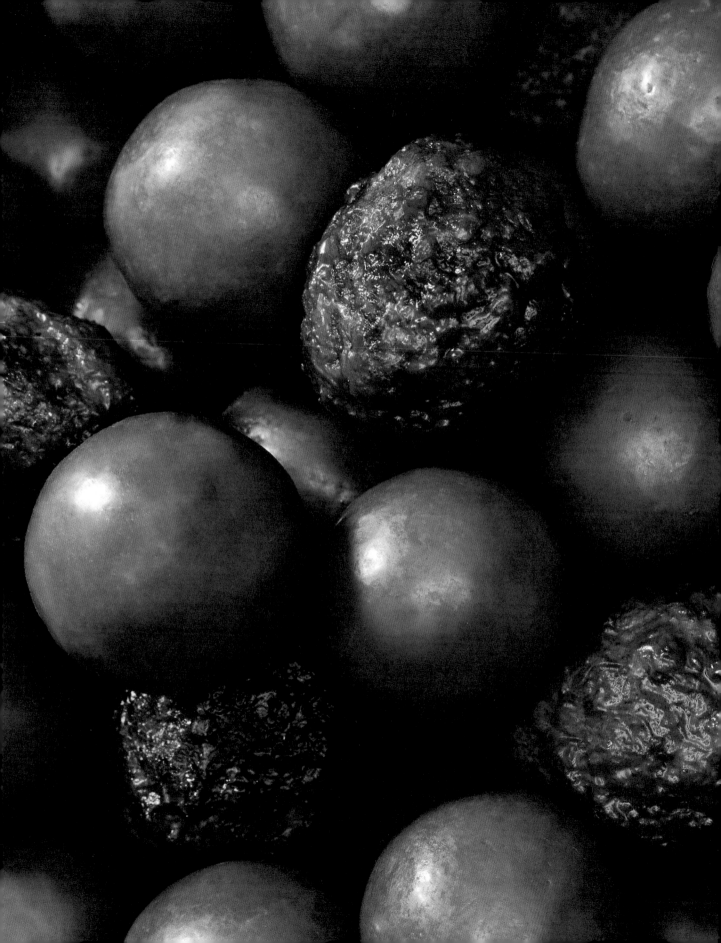

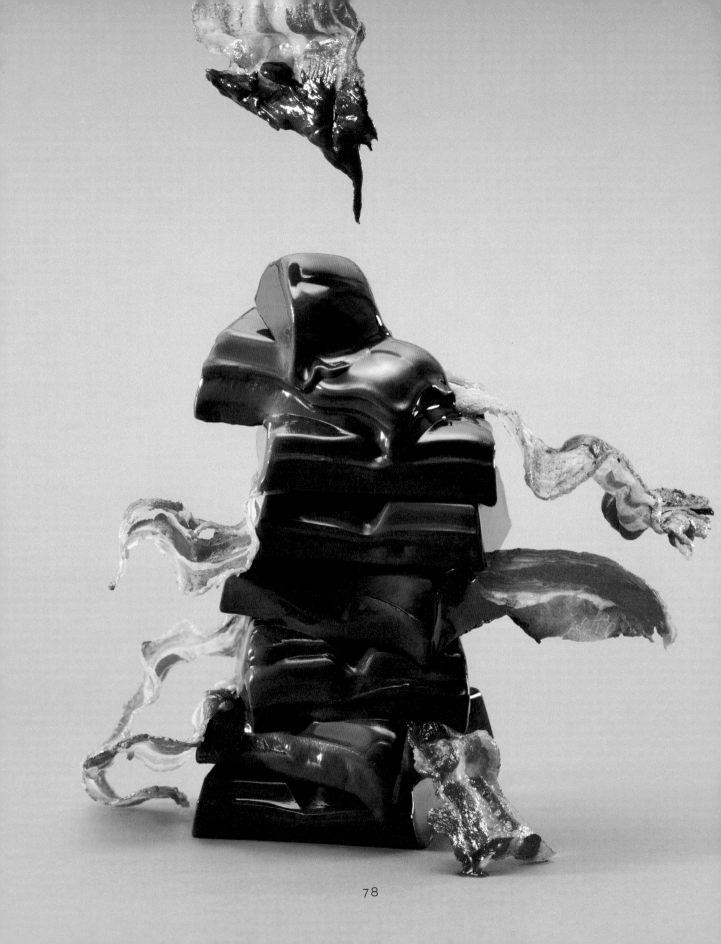

Chocolate Bacon

Ingredients

Bacon

Milk Chocolate

You don't have to be pregnant to appreciate this delicacy. Because bacon. And chocolate. But also bacon.

When I first heard about this craving I thought this shouldn't only be for pregnant women. I soon realized that this has been a thing in the US for years, and for obvious reasons, because bacon goes well with everything.

Now imagine it with chocolate. Few things in the universe complement each other better than chocolate and bacon. Rainbows and unicorns do, but their taste is supposed to be a bit bland.

Fry yourself some bacon until it's nice and crisp. Let it cool, and dab off the grease. Melt some milk chocolate and cover your bacon in it. Make sure the bacon is dry and crispy before you completely cover it with chocolate, because soft, moist bacon isn't really bacon.

Week 31

Your baby is now the size of a Pineapple. Not great with Mustard, or is it?

Pockethoney

Ingredients

A box of
Honey Mustard tubes

A large sweater or pants

This recipe is endless satisfaction as it calls for no preparation, plates, or patience.
A crazy snack leaving no evidence is exactly what you need by now. Another advantage is you can buy it in bulk and eat it like that too. Honey Mustard. In a tube. Or two. Or a box. Whatever, the point is to eat it pure. Straight out of the tube. Empty the sucker.

The very best part of this strange snack is that you can do it without shame because what a man can't see a man can't judge. Sneak the tube in your sleeve anywhere you want and have a quick treat when no one is looking
At your inlaws in between the first and second course of the christmas dinner for example.
In the waiting room of your gynaecologist.
Or empty the tube on the tube.

This will be your honey. Mustard.

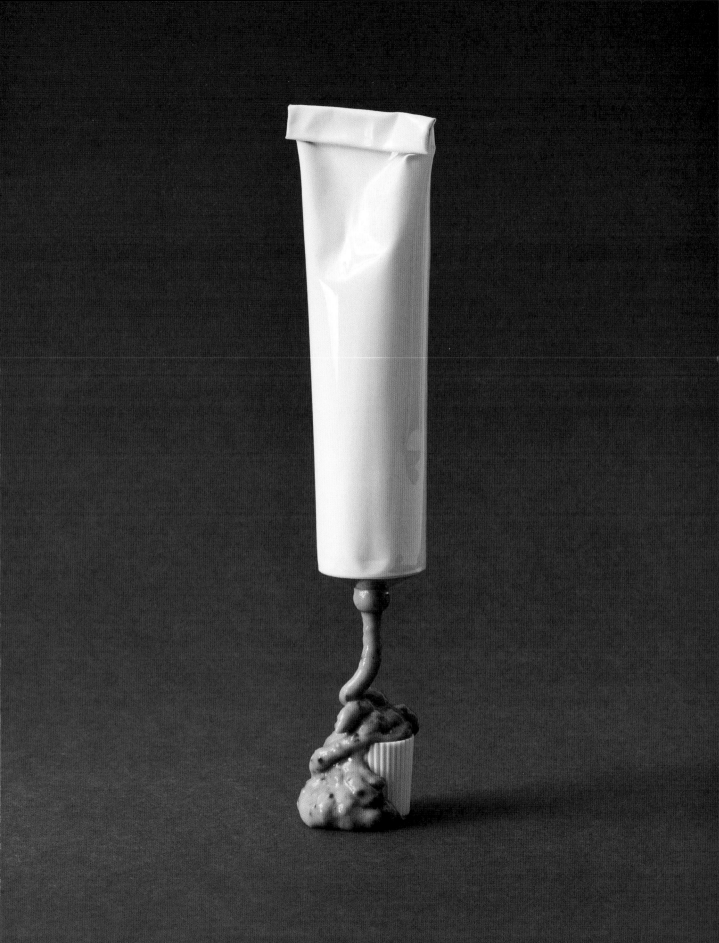

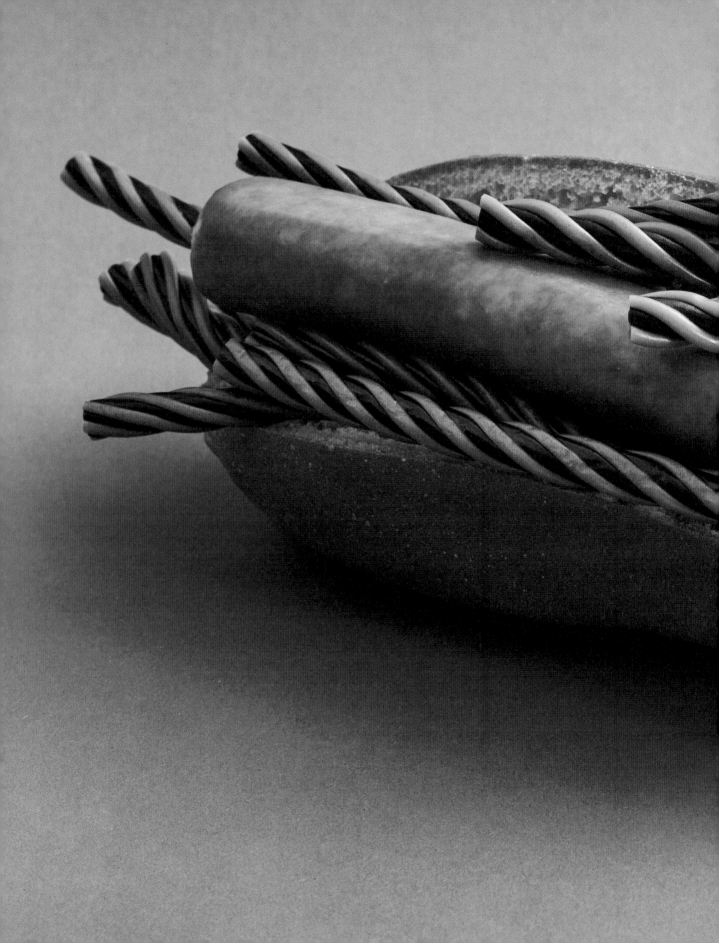

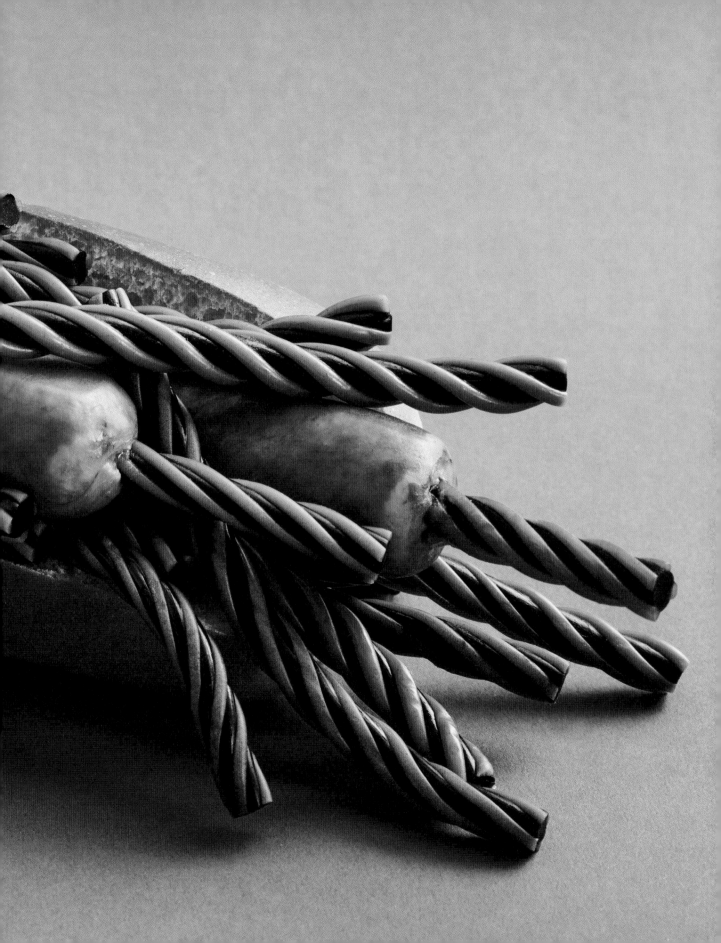

Morndog Liquor

Week 32

Your baby now weighs about 1.7 kg, approximately the weight of 17 Hot Dogs.

Ingredients

Hot dogs

Liquorice

Buns, corn or regular

Onion

Mustard

Ketchup

Crispy Fried Onions

This is as close as you will get to liquor for a very long time. Liquorice. On a hot dog. Right when you wake up. The sooner the better as it will help you overcome your morning sickness. Unlike actual liquor, liquorice isn't that harmful to your body and baby, however you should pace yourself as liquorice drives your blood pressure up faster than your know-it-all cousin Jenny.

Like becoming pregnant it's all about timing, you need to make sure you have a well-oiled machine waiting for you in the morning. This can either be through the labour of your significant other or you can prep it yourself. Put your grill pan out on the stove the evening before. Cut some onions and pickles, get your sauerkraut ready, and put all of them in the fridge, except for your buns. No one likes a cold bun. Go to bed with the promise of hot dogs in the morning.

Once awake, go to your kitchen and, depending on your wieners, boil or grill them for six to eight minutes and toast your buns. After they're toasted, put some mustard, ketchup, onions, pickles, sauerkraut, and liquorice on your bun. Then your wiener, more condiments, and top it off with crispy fried onions. Eat this! That will teach your nausea a lesson.

Week 33

Your baby is now approximately as tall as a 43 cm stack of Brownies.

Dijon Brownie

Ingredients

Brownie

Dijon Mustard

Ever since its invention in the late 19th century in the US, the brownie has conquered hearts around the world. It even got a place in the bucket of a certain famous ice cream brand, more than once. People eat it hot, cold, even uncooked. Yet to some, it's still not good enough. They prefer it with a little kick.

The pregnant heart is incomparable when it comes to flavour and when it tells you to drown your brownie in Dijon mustard, you do it. I'm quite certain that, unlike some other recipes, this one is a pregnancy exclusive. Few have the heart or the stomach to add this French twist to an all-time American classic.

But if you do, there are a couple of ways you can go about it. You can follow your own batter recipe, stir the Dijon mustard into it and eat it raw. You can cook your own mustard infused brownie and top it off with a spoonful. If you're not much of a culinary prodigy, you can always pick up some brownies at a bakery or supermarket and dip it in your mustard jar. Whichever way you choose, you'll have them all to yourself. Guaranteed.

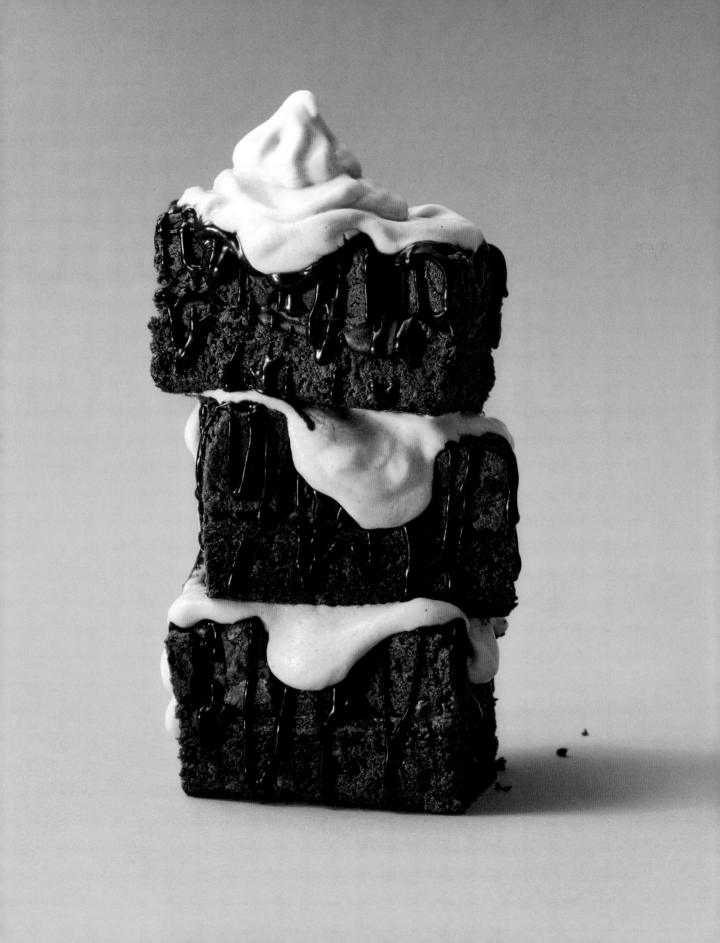

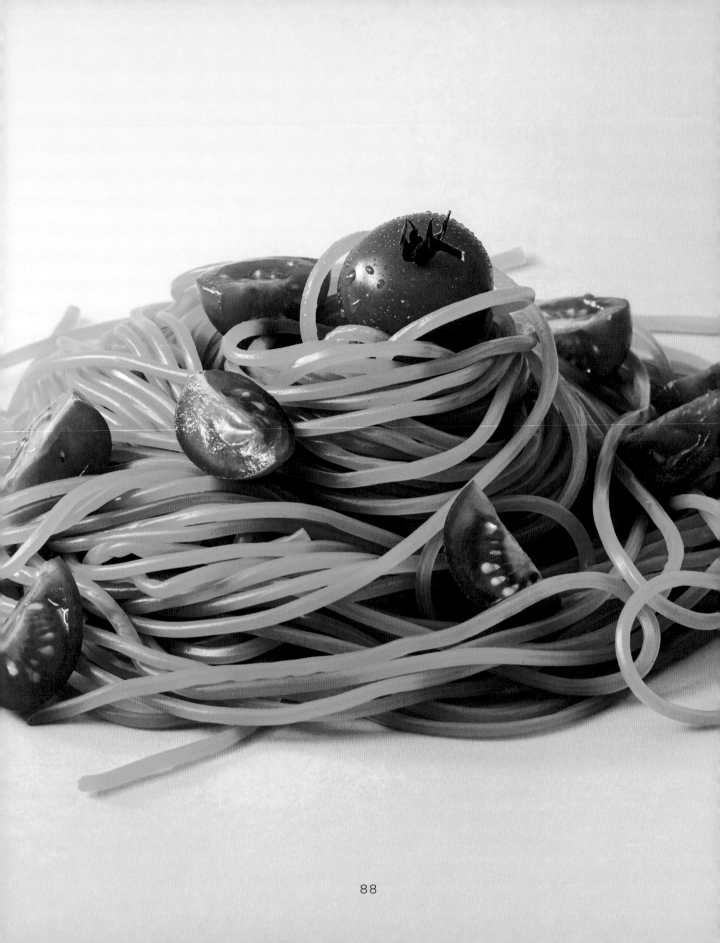

Candy Pomodori

Ingredients

Cherry Tomatoes

Apple Candy Laces

Candy and vegetables. Arch enemies in the world of children, just another recipe filled with delicious contrast in the world of moms-to-be. Sweetness of tomato combined with sourness of green apple candy laces. Even the colours are the pinnacle of contrast as red and green are direct opposites in the world of colour.

Sometimes it's not just the flavour; texture and looks can have a tremendous attractive power when it comes to appetite. This recipe pulls all the triggers of pregnancy cravings, flavour, texture, ease, and looks. The simplicity in this dish is its true strength: only two ingredients and yet so much to offer. In this particular recipe less truly ís more.

Your baby now weighs about the same as a 2.3 kg jar of Peanut Butter.

Peanut Butter Jelly Time

Ingredients

Cheap, Fresh Bread

Peanut Butter

Strawberry Jam or Jelly

A timeless dish. Really it is. You'll keep making this dish for years after your pregnancy. Not necessarily for yourself, because your equally addicted offspring will crave it, and guess who'll have to make it.

Get some regular white bread. Nothing fancy: the cheaper ones tend to work best, just make sure it's fresh. Grab two slices and spread one with a thick layer of peanut butter and the other with an equally generous coating of strawberry jelly or jam. Put the two together and apply pressure so the filling almost oozes out of the sides. Stack and repeat until your sandwich has reached the height of your dreams.

Now it's time to get rid of that nasty crust. A crust on a PBJ sandwich is like the sleazy uncle who ruins your birthday parties, so let's not invite him. Slice it right off, unveiling a sandwich layered like a birthday cake.

IT'S PEANUT BUTTER JELLY TIME!

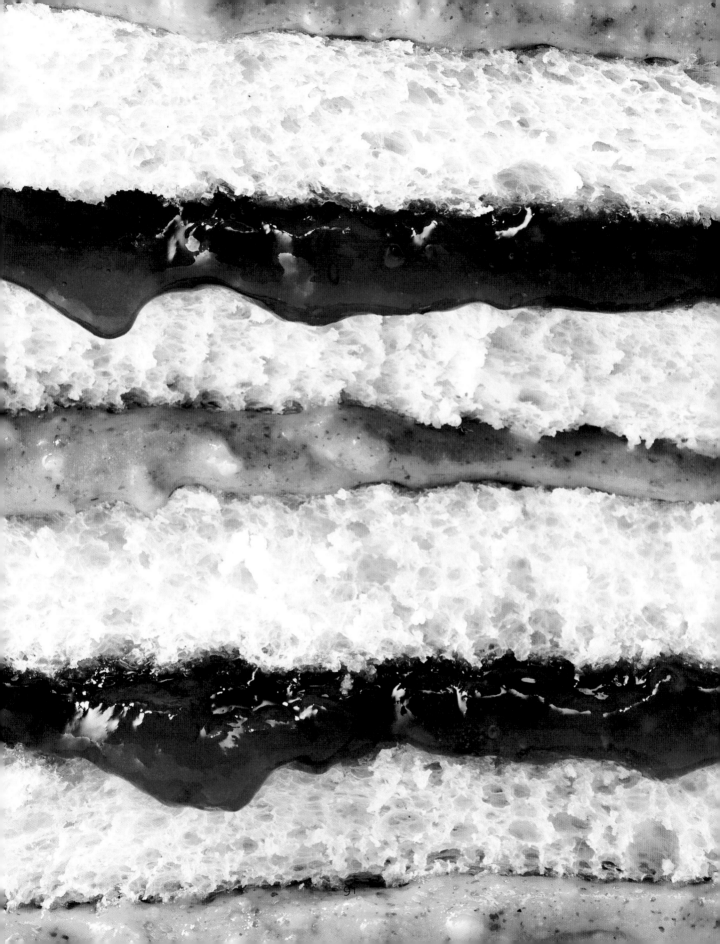

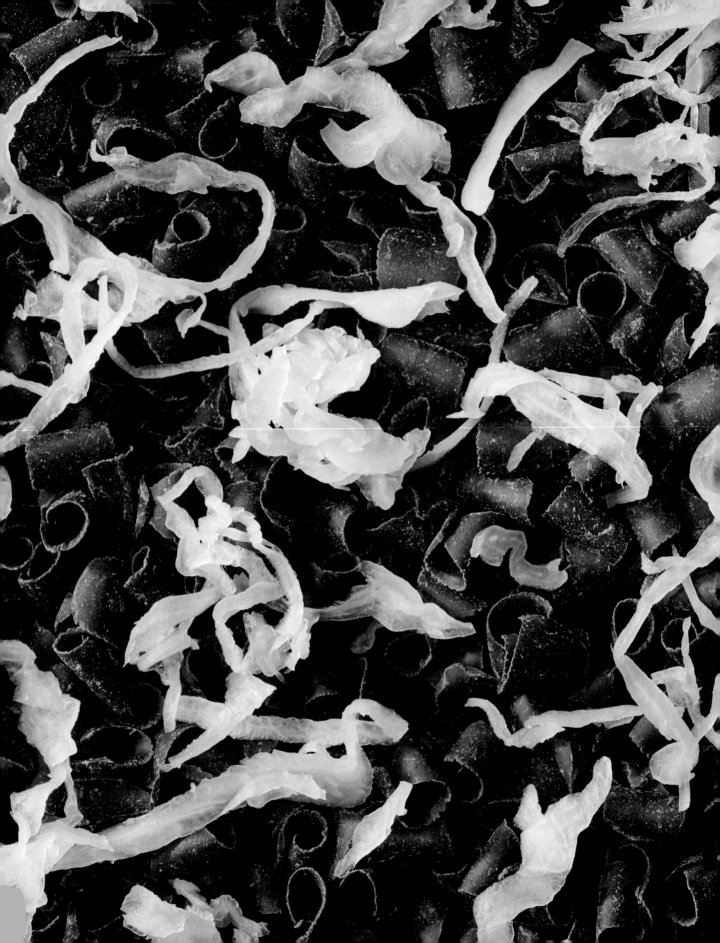

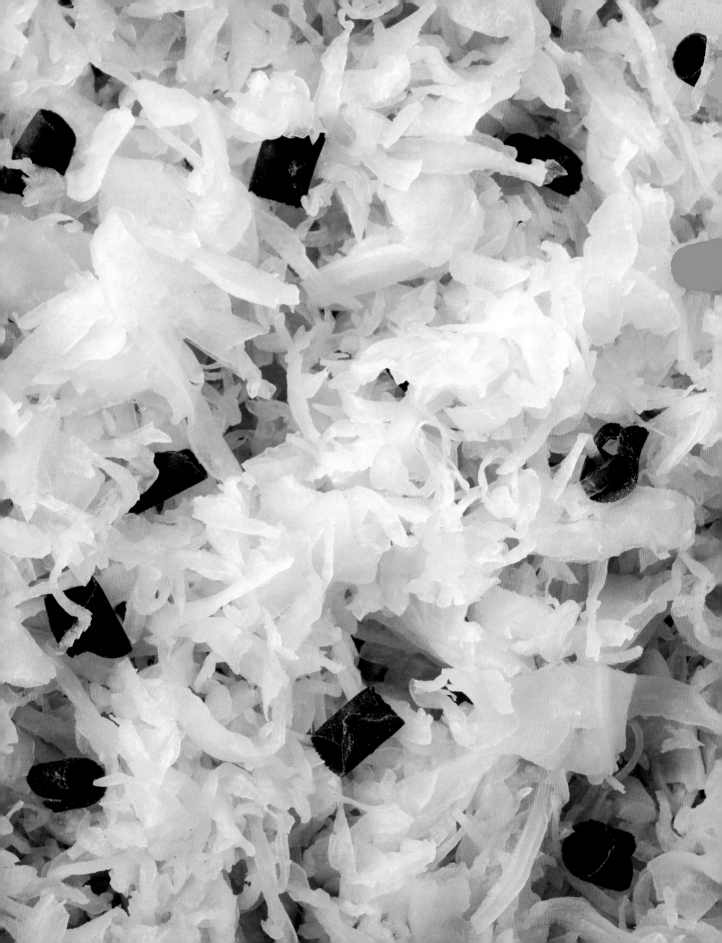

Strac
cia
tella
Kraut

Your baby now weighs as much as a 2.6 kg serving of Stracciatella Kraut.

Ingredients

Sauerkraut

Tony Chocolonely
Salted Caramel

Das germanische gericht with *schokolade* in it. Sauerkraut and chocolate. If there was anything that brought depression and despair when I was a boy, it was a plate of this stuff. Sauerkraut, not chocolate, to be clear. No matter how many marbles I had won, or tricks I learned on my rollerblades, this dish was singlehandedly able to crush all the joy out of my life in one plate. Yet one little boy's hell can be another pregnant woman's heaven. Especially if you hide some chocolate in there.

Take your sauerkraut out of the package and drain it in a strainer. Wash off the brine with water thoroughly, unless you prefer the sharp salty taste of the brine. Put it in a pot and just cover it in water. When the water boils put on the lid and put the heat on the lowest setting, let it boil for about 30-40 minutes. Take it out and drain it again. Now here's some room for creativity, you can balance your chocolate nine-to-one to the sauerkraut or the other way around. Stir the chocolate through the kraut or add it when you serve it.

Although anything can be great with chocolate, I would never surrender to Sauerkraut. Not even with Tony Chocolonely's Salted Caaramel in there. Okay maybe.

Brownie Batter

Ingredients

1/2 cup of melted Butter

1 cup of Sugar

A pinch of Salt

2 Eggs

1/3 cup of Cocoa

1/2 cup of Flour

1/4 teaspoon Baking Powder

Like stated before in the Dijon Brownie recipe, people go crazy for brownies. So crazy even, some want to eat it before it is baked. But it is not just flavour and texture, it's the speed of this treat that get the saliva glands going here.

This is a recipe for the impatient ones. The ones that don't have the patience to wait twenty-five minutes for their snack. If you fit into this categorie, I predict agony. Because those nine months your little nacho is in the oven are going to feel endless. You can't buy your batter off the shelf in a supermarket, like you can with cooked brownies, so it will need a little work. Mix half a cup of melted butter with a cup of sugar, a pinch of salt, two eggs, one-third cup of cocoa, half a cup of flour, and baking powder. Stir it until smooth and then lick it until clean.

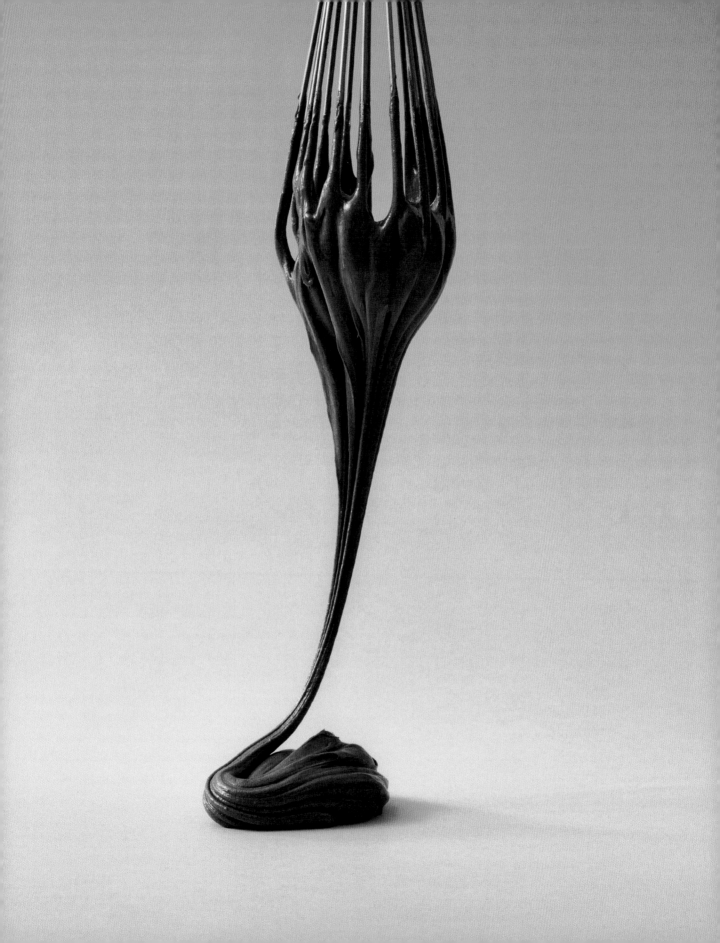

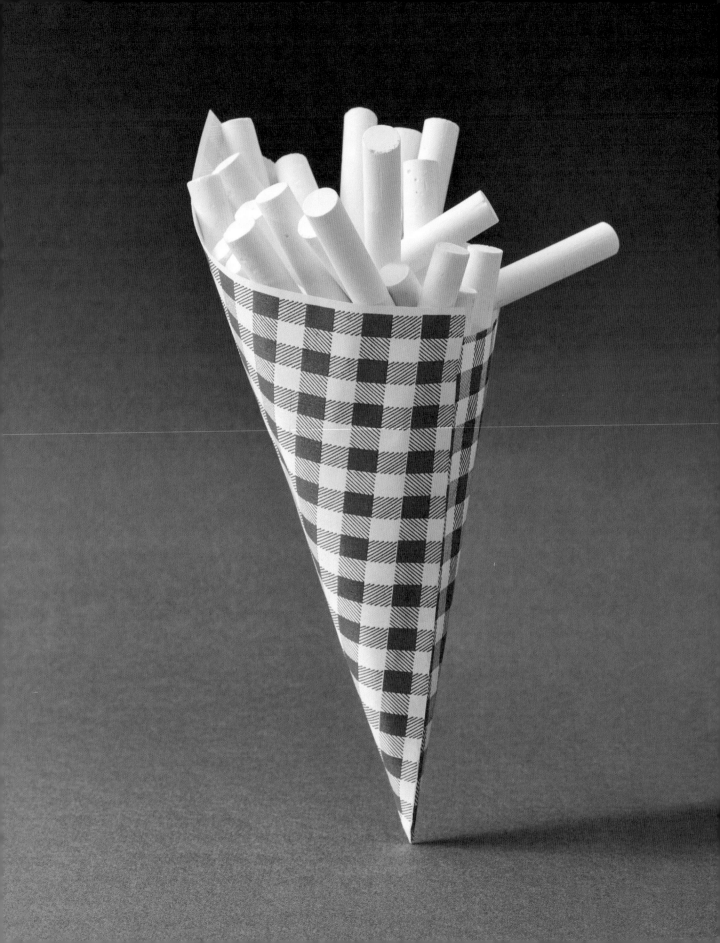

Drywall Delux

Ingredients

Remodelled rooms

Fresh drywall

Chalk

Dirt

Plaster

Some women have cravings so bad no food can satisfy their hunger. They have an appetite for something with a little more substance. Drywall, chalk, plaster, or concrete — you know, the stuff you build houses with.

If your tastebuds are already tingling and your salivary glands are wetting your tongue while reading this, beware. You are in a state you could eat through the walls of your newly furbished nursery, which, although satisfying, is a very bad idea. You have a condition called pica and you should get in touch with a doctor or pregnancy professional.

STOP looking at the wall as if it's a stack of blueberry pancakes. It's not. It's a supporting wall of your house.

Hot Melons

Ingredients

Watermelon

Tabasco

Watermelon and tabasco. I am truly amazed how such random things can really hit the sweet spot. Or in this case the spicy spot.

I've heard lots of spicy food cravings but always in combination with a certain predictable food combo. Watermelons do not fit this exact category for me, but it left me wondering if the wateriness of the melon would cancel out the fieriness of the Tabasco. I can assure you it does not. Personally I'm not a fan of Tabasco or watermelon, but I think some of you had their mouths water at watermelon.

It's another simple recipe that you can customise to your liking, so go for it. Let it hit your spicy spot. Use with caution though: remember it has to come out, too.

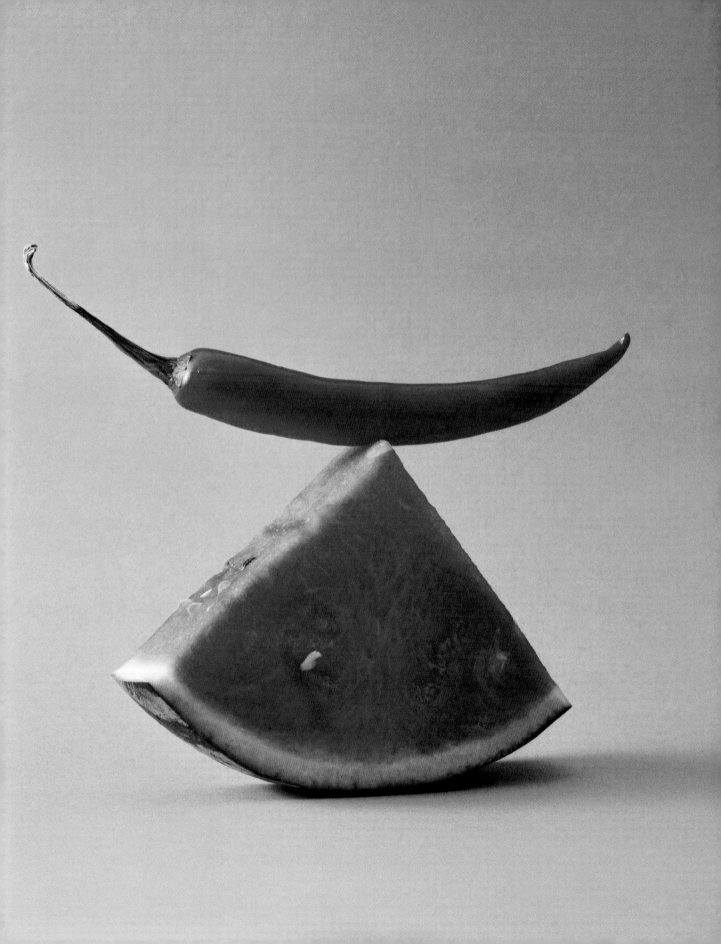

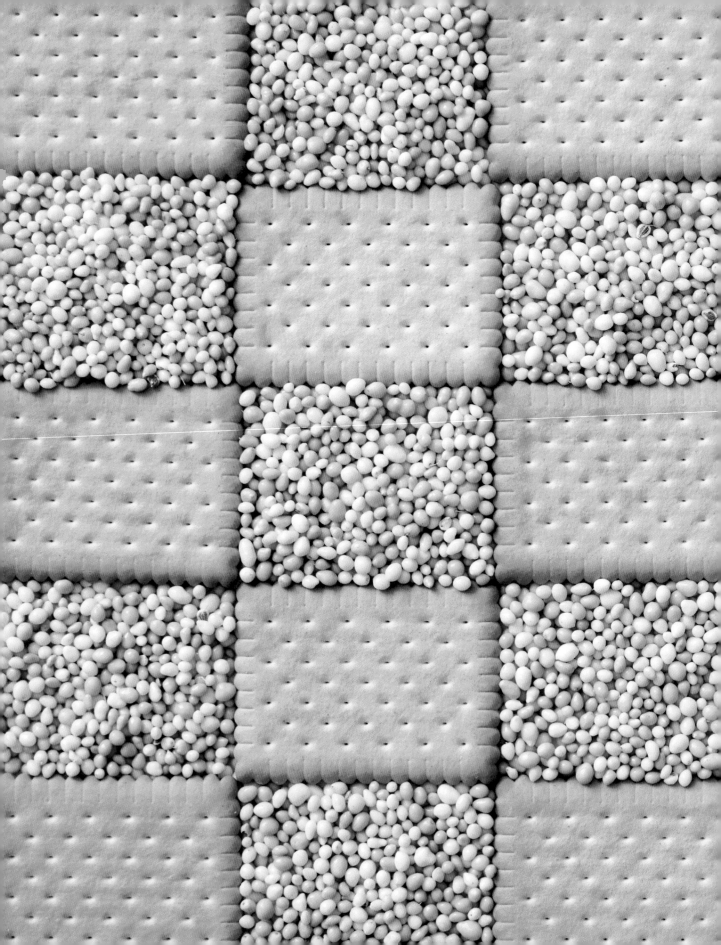

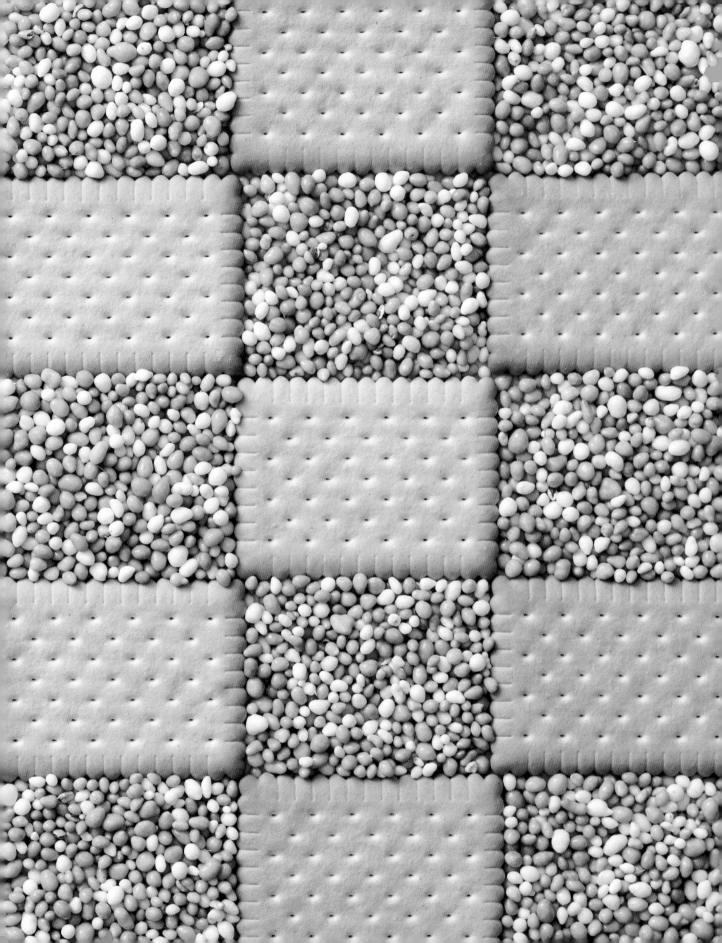

Biscuits. with Mice

Ingredients

Biscuits

Coloured Mice

This last one just sounds weird, but it's actually a festive treat for the whole family after you've given birth. Biscuits with mice.

I'm Dutch and in The Netherlands it's a tradition to eat *'Beschuit'* biscuits or rusk sprinkled with mice to celebrate the newest member of the family. Blue mice for a boy, pink if it's a girl.

These mice aren't the mice your cat drags in, but are made out of anise and are more like sprinkles. It's very common here to eat sprinkles on a sandwich or biscuits so for such a special occasion someone thought it would be a great idea to give it it's own kind of sprinkles. But from all the reactions I have gotten in my life from my foreign friends for eating a sandwich or biscuit with sprinkles, I guess it might not be so ordinary after all. Congratulations with your new child! Or as we say it: *Gefeliciteerd!*

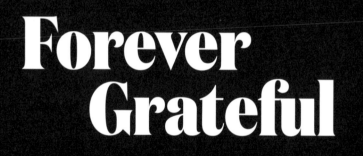

This book has been in the making since 2014 and boy has it been a delivery. Unlike a regular pregnancy this baby took 240 weeks to be delivered. And I couldn't have done it if it weren't for a few extraordinary people.

I would like to start with the biggest inspirations: all the pregnant women and their strange appetites I've encountered in my life. Most of you will know who you are but a few I want to name specifically, mainly the strain of cheese lovers that is my family. My mother and her appetite for Brie and my sister and her appetite for almost every kind of cheese.

Rene Mesman for the stunning photography, Claartje Lindhout for the both mouth-watering and gut-wrenching dishes, and both for their brilliant creative collaboration in shaping these dishes. Luminous-ci for the incredible image quality and retouching. Dennis van Gaalen en Eline Wieriks for their keen eye for design and supporting me in meeting the print deadline. John Loughlin for ensuring there was not a single unintended denglish phrase in there. Bionda Dias and Sara van de Ven for seeing the beauty in this disgusting idea and deciding to publish it regardless.

All the friends that encouraged me, but in particular my friends Dick Buschman and Délia Lauret for inspiring me to take the first steps in making this book. My friend Perre van den Brink for pushing me to actually visit a publisher and try to finish it.

And last but definitely not least my incredible girlfriend Amé Maassen for motivating and encouraging me to keep on going, for supporting me through all the weekends and late nights, and for her empowering words in the stressful periods.

I could not have done it without you.

Find your
crave quickly

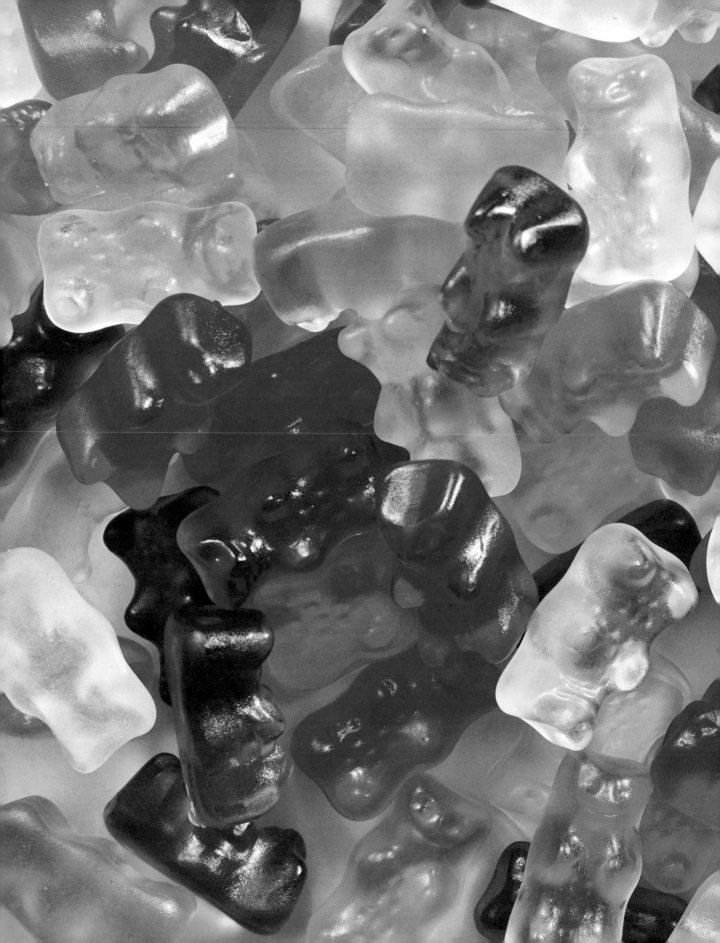